*The right diet is a powerful weapon
in the war against cancer!*

- The foods you should eat to help prevent cancer—and the foods you should avoid
- The remarkable benefits of a high-fiber diet
- How to prepare and store foods to best lock in their cancer-fighting nutrients
- The facts on flavonoids—and how to get more of them into your diet
- The latest findings on soy and its value as a breast cancer preventative
- Why tomatoes and tomato products are good for you—and should be eaten at least twice a week
- Daily meal plans, recipes . . . AND MORE!

The information included in
FOODS THAT COMBAT CANCER
is your frontline defense providing important
strategies to help you enjoy a healthy, long life!

Foods That
COMBAT
CANCER

The Nutritional Way to Wellness

Maggie Greenwood-Robinson, Ph.D.

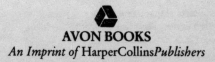

AVON BOOKS
An Imprint of HarperCollinsPublishers

AVON BOOKS
An Imprint of HarperCollins*Publishers*
10 East 53rd Street
New York, New York 10022-5299

First Avon Books paperback printing: June 2003

Avon Trademark Reg. U.S. Pat. Off. and in Other Countries, Marca Registrada, Hecho en U.S.A.
HarperCollins ® is a trademark of HarperCollins Publishers Inc.

Printed in the U.S.A.

10 9 8 7 6 5

ACKNOWLEDGMENTS

Special thanks to the following people for their work and contributions to this book: my agent Madeleine Morel, 2M Communications, Ltd.; Lynn Sonberg of Lynn Sonberg Books; the staff at Avon Books; and my husband Jeff, for love and patience during the research and writing of this book.

CONTENTS

Foods That
COMBAT
CANCER

INTRODUCTION

If you're like most people, you know someone whose life has been affected by cancer. So feared is this disease that some are afraid to even utter its name, calling it instead the "Big C."

Right now, more than 560,000 Americans a year lose their lives to cancer, and an estimated 1.2 million new cases are diagnosed annually. It is the second-leading cause of death in the United States.

But let's not dwell on the negatives. Did you know that cancer is now considered a *preventable* disease?

Based on a major research project into the link between cancer and diet, the American Institute for Cancer Research (AICR) estimates that 375,000 cases of cancer could be prevented every year in the United States if we made better dietary choices.

But to make the right dietary adjustments, you need to know which foods contain which cancer-fighting nutrients—information that until now hasn't been easy to find in one easy-to-use quick reference. *Foods That*

Combat Cancer changes all that. It tells health-conscious consumers, as well as cancer survivors, what they need to know in a comprehensive, user-friendly format. Here you will find more than 2,000 brand-name and basic food items and the cancer-fighting nutrients found in each one, based on serving size.

In addition, you'll learn how to identify the freshest foods, store and prepare foods to lock in their nutrients, and plan your daily diet for maximum cancer protection. Also included are three full days of menus, complete with easy-to-prepare recipes.

So if you're ready to hedge your bets against cancer, *Foods That Combat Cancer* will show you how.

CHAPTER 1

RESIST CANCER NOW

～

Consider: Nearly 70 percent of all cancer—one of the most dreaded diseases known to humanity—is linked to poor diet. What this rather startling statistic means is you can slash your odds of getting the disease by what you put on your plate! And it doesn't take a grit-your-teeth-and-do-it dietary commitment, either.

In fact, the American Institute for Cancer Research (AICR) says a simple change like eating five servings of fruits and vegetables a day will cut your cancer risk by more than 20 percent. And get this: Some of the most protective fruits and vegetables are those we eat most often, including carrots, onions, garlic, broccoli, green vegetables, tomatoes, citrus fruits, and legumes. That's the conclusion of a major review study, published in the *Journal of the American Dietetic Association,* which analyzed more than 200 other cancer-diet studies. As you plan your diet to include more of these foods, you can use this counter to easily identify the richest sources of cancer-fighting substances in fruits, vegetables, and other foods.

Along with eating more fruits and vegetables, there are other incredibly easy ways to roll back your risk—things most of us should be doing but aren't—like reducing our fat intake and eating more fiber. According to Ritva Butrum, Ph.D., vice president for research at AICR, "Future cancer-fighting efforts are more likely to revolve around dietary adjustments than miracle pills."

That position is supported by hundreds of studies looking into the relationship between cancer and diet—studies that strongly support the fact that cancer is preventable through diet. For a synopsis of which foods are the most protective against specific types of cancers, refer to the table below.

FOODS THAT PROTECT AGAINST CANCER

Cancers	Potentially Protective Foods
Bladder	Garlic, green leafy vegetables, soy foods, tea,* yellow/orange vegetables, yogurt and other fermented milk products
Breast	1% milk, apples, bran, Brazil nuts, beans and legumes, broccoli, Brussels sprouts, button and shiitake mushrooms, cabbage, carrots and carrot juice, cherries, fattier fish (salmon, tuna), flaxseeds, flaxseed oil (high-lignan), garlic, kohlrabi, lowfat dairy products (with the exception of skim milk), nuts, olive oil, radishes, soy foods, spinach, whole grains, yellow/orange vegetables, yogurt
Cervical	Romaine lettuce and other green leafy vegetables, tomatoes and tomato products, yellow/orange vegetables
Colon	Brazil nuts, broccoli, Brussels sprouts, cabbage, carrots, cauliflower, celery, fattier fish, garlic, grapes and grape juice, kale, legumes, lettuce, lowfat dairy products, nuts, oat bran, oranges and orange juice, spinach, tomatoes and tomato products, wheat bran, whole grains, yogurt and other fermented milk products
Endometrial	Broccoli, Brussels sprouts, cabbage, cauliflower, kale and other green leafy vegetables, yellow/orange vegetables

Cancers	Potentially Protective Foods
Esophageal	Green tea, tomatoes and tomato products
Kidney	Tea
Leukemia	Tea
Liver	Garlic, green tea
Lung	Brazil nuts, broccoli, Brussels sprouts, cabbage, carrots and other yellow/orange vegetables, cauliflower, hot peppers, kale, lowfat dairy products (with the exception of skim milk), onions, oranges, spinach and other green leafy vegetables, tomatoes and tomato products
Oral	Tomatoes and tomato products
Ovarian	Broccoli, Brussels sprouts, cabbage, cauliflower, kale and other green leafy vegetables, yellow/orange vegetables
Pancreatic	Legumes, tea, tomatoes and tomato products
Prostate	Brazil nuts, Brussels sprouts, broccoli, cabbage, canola oil, cauliflower, kale, lowfat dairy products (with the exception of skim milk), olive oil, peanut oil, soy foods, tomatoes and tomato products
Stomach	Broccoli, Brussels sprouts, cabbage, cauliflower, fava beans, garlic, green tea, kale, onions, oranges and other citrus fruits, tomatoes and tomato products, whole grains

*All tea referred to in this chart is either green or black, not herbal tea.

More good news: If you stay active, maintain a healthy weight, don't smoke, and *continue to eat right*, your risk shrinks even more—by nearly 70 percent.

With this in mind, let's take a closer look at how you can reduce the threat of cancer by tweaking your diet, in some very easy ways, starting now.

Dietary Fat

Diets overloaded with two types of fat—*saturated fats* and *trans-fats*—have been implicated in the development of prostate cancer, colon cancer, and quite possibly, breast cancer. Saturated fats are present predominantly in animal foods, specifically red meat and animal fat. Trans-fats are synthetic fats that act like saturated fats in the body and are found in stick margarine and short-ening. Trans-fats are produced when vegetable fats are converted from liquid to solid form in a process known as hydrogenation. The problem with trans-fats is that, once in the body, they inflict damage to cell mem-branes, making cells indefensible to invaders.

Saturated Fat and Cancer

A slew of studies has found a strong link between saturated fat and prostate cancer, the deadliest cancer among American men. Saturated fat is thought to alter levels of sex hormones, creating an internal environ-ment that can promote this form of cancer. In a study conducted in France, investigators found that men whose diets contained more than 30 to 40 percent fat (most of it saturated) had a higher risk of developing prostate cancer than men whose diets contained less than 30 percent fat.

The risk of colon cancer catching up with you some time in the future may also be related to the amount of saturated fat you eat. A Harvard study discovered that men who ate low amounts of saturated fat (7 percent of their calories) had half the rate of precancerous polyps of men who ate double that amount (14 per-cent). Polyps can progress into tumors in the colon. A diet high in red meat—a major source of saturated fat—has also been implicated in a higher risk of colon cancer.

Breast cancer is the most extensively studied cancer in terms of its relationship to dietary fat. But until fairly recently, saturated fat was believed to be a crim-inal in the promotion of breast cancer. However, a study of nearly 90,000 women conducted by doctors at Boston's Brigham and Women's Hospital exonerated saturated fat, finding little evidence of the suspected breast cancer link. Other research has produced similar findings. Most investigators believe that multiple factors are at work to increase the risk of breast cancer—including genetics, menstrual history, physical activity, body fat, and overall diet—so it's difficult to pin the cause on saturated fat alone.

Trans-Fats and Cancer

Trans-fats, however, have been blamed for an increased risk of breast cancer. A University of North Carolina study discovered that women whose fatty tissue contained high levels of trans-fats and low levels of healthier vegetable-based fats were three times more likely to develop breast cancer. Other research has found that diets high in trans-fats are also associated with prostate cancer.

Anti-Cancer Fats

As for the type of fat you eat, oil from fish has been found to be protective against some cancers, in contrast to the possible cancer-promoting effect of saturated fat. What's more, in countries where people eat a lot of olive oil, rates of breast cancer and colon cancer are very low.

What You Can Do Now

The American Institute for Cancer Research and other leading health organizations recommend that you reduce your fat intake to 20 percent or less of your total daily calories. On a 2,000-calorie-a-day diet, that equates to about 44 grams of fat daily. Less than 10 grams of that daily fat allotment should come from saturated fat. Here are some easy ways to reduce the fat in your diet:

- Use this counter to pinpoint which foods contain an excess of unhealthy fats and then shun those foods. (The lower the number of fat grams in a serving, the better.)
- Stick to lowfat and nonfat food choices: lean proteins like white meat poultry, fish, and egg whites; lowfat dairy products; lowfat salad dressings; and other reduced-fat foods.
- Cut the fat from your diet by making healthful substitutions. For example: a baked potato for French fries; lowfat milk for whole milk; plain yogurt for sour cream or mayonnaise; ice milk or frozen yogurt for ice cream; a grilled chicken sandwich for a cheeseburger; fat-free pretzels for potato chips, to name just a few lower-fat substitutions.
- Broil, bake, or microwave foods rather than frying them.
- Remove skin from chicken prior to cooking.
- Watch out for "hidden" fat in certain foods too. Fat is added to crackers, cookies, breads, and rolls. You may not see it, but it's there.
- Read food labels. Even foods claiming to be lowfat or natural may contain trans-fats. That being so, avoid food products that have the words "hydrogenated" or "partially hydrogenated" on their labels. Hydrogenated fats contain trans-fats.
- Limit or avoid using stick margarine, which is the most highly hydrogenated fat of all. Softer tub and liquid margarines are lower in trans-fats, and

are a better alternative. Or, check out the new "trans-free" margarines made without trans-fats.

- Avoid cooking with stick margarine or shortening. Substitute vegetable oil. Or, for a fat-free recipe, replace the fat with applesauce or fruit puree.
- Choose margarines and other fats that contain liquid vegetable oil as the first ingredient and no more than two grams of saturated fat per tablespoon.
- Cut back on foods that are fried in vegetable shortening, such as French fries or fried chicken.
- Use olive oil in place of margarine—for dipping breads, rolls, or bagels.
- Use olive oil or canola oil to sauté vegetables and other foods.

Fiber

Every time you crunch down on a piece of celery or bite into an apple, you're eating fiber, an indigestible but indispensable remnant of food. Low amounts of fiber in the diet are linked to dozens of medical problems, and cancer is just one of them.

An ever-growing body of research suggests that you can reduce your odds of getting cancer by increasing your fiber intake. Here are several recent examples:

- In June 2001, results from the largest-ever study into diet and cancer (testing 400,000 people from nine countries over 15 years), called the European Prospective Investigation of Cancer and Nutrition, found that people who ate the most fiber reduced their risk of colon cancer by up to 40 percent.

- A March 2001 study reported that eating cereal fiber lowers the risk of stomach cancer by 60 percent.
- A February 2001 study reported that people who eat plenty of fiber foods have about half the risk of cancers of the mouth and throat.

These are just a few of the many studies showing the importance of fiber in reducing your cancer risk. The key is to populate your diet with more high-fiber foods. Some of your best fiber bets from various food groups are listed below. In addition, you'll find a vast array of other high-fiber foods in the counter. Look for them mostly among vegetables, fruits, cereals, grains, and nuts and seeds.

Food	Serving Size	Fiber Content (gm)
Beans & Legumes		
Beans, kidney, red, canned	½ cup	8
Peas, split, boiled	½ cup	8
Lentils, boiled	½ cup	8
Beans, black, boiled	½ cup	7.5
Beans, pinto, boiled	½ cup	7.5
Refried beans, canned	½ cup	6.5
Lima beans, boiled	½ cup	6.5
Beans, kidney, red, boiled	½ cup	6.5
Beans, baked, canned, plain or vegetarian	½ cup	6.5
Beans, white, canned	½ cup	6.5
Vegetables (Other)		
Artichokes, boiled	1 cup	9
Peas, boiled	1 cup	9

Food	Serving Size	Fiber Content (gm)
Vegetables, mixed, boiled	1 cup	8
Lettuce, iceberg	1 head	7.5
Pumpkin, canned	1 cup	7
Peas, canned	1 cup	7
Artichoke, boiled	1 medium	6.5
Brussels sprouts, frozen, boiled	1 cup	6
Parsnips, boiled	1 cup	6
Sauerkraut, canned	1 cup	6
Cereals, Grains & Pasta		
All-Bran with Extra Fiber (Kellogg's)	½ cup	15
Fiber One (General Mills)	½ cup	14
Granola, homemade	1 cup	13
All-Bran (Kellogg's)	½ cup	9.7
Bulgur wheat, cooked	1 cup	8
Raisin Bran (Kellogg's)	1 cup	8
100% Bran (Post)	⅓ cup	8.3
Bran Chex (Kellogg's)	1 cup	8
Shredded Wheat and Bran	1¼ cups	8
Oat bran, cooked	½ cup	6
Fruits		
Avocado, Florida	1 avocado	18
Raspberries, frozen, unsweetened	1 cup	17
Prunes, stewed	1 cup	16
Dates, chopped	1 cup	13
Pears, dried	10 halves	13
Avocado, California	1 avocado	8.7
Raspberries, raw	1 cup	8
Blueberries, raw	1 cup	7.6
Papaya, whole	1 fruit	5.5
Figs, dried	2 figs	4.6

Source: Nutrient Data Laboratory. USDA Nutrient Database for Standard Reference, Release 14. Beltsville, Maryland.

What You Can Do Now

The National Research Council recommends 20 to 35 grams of fiber a day from a variety of plant sources. Most Americans get only about 11 grams a day, however.

Here are some tips for increasing your fiber intake:

- Read labels. To qualify as a good source of fiber, food should contain at least 2.5 to 3 grams. In addition, the counter can help you find high-fiber foods that fill this bill.
- Make high-fiber substitutions: brown rice for white, whole grain cereals for processed cereals, a bran muffin for a doughnut, bean dips for sour cream dips, black beans or kidney beans for ground beef, and so forth.
- Snack on fruits, dried fruits, or raw vegetables, rather than on potato chips or candy.
- Add beans and other legumes to soups and extra beans to chili.
- Purchase packaged cereals that have been fortified with extra fiber.
- Sprinkle your cereal with a few tablespoons of raw wheat bran.
- Eat unpeeled fruit such as apples or pears.

Flavonoids

Packing a wallop of power against cancer are a group of natural substances called flavonoids, found abundantly in fruits, vegetables, grains, tea, and wine. More than 5,000 flavonoids have been discovered in nature, and many are responsible for the bright colors of the fruits and vegetables you eat. Flavonoids are also essential for the proper absorption of vitamin C, one of the most important antioxidants and cancer fighters. In fact, flavonoids are what make natural vitamin C (found in foods) more effective than synthetic supplemental vitamin C, by improving and prolonging the function of the vitamin.

Some of the more familiar flavonoids are catechins, citrin, hesperidin, quercetin, and rutin. Of these, catechins and quercetin have been the best studied for their protection against cancer.

Catechins are abundant in green and black teas, red wine, and chocolate. Research with animals shows that catechins inhibit cancers of most major organs: skin, lungs, esophagus, stomach, liver, small intestine, colon, pancreas, bladder, and mammary glands. In humans, studies in Japan and China hint that drinking green tea is associated with a reduced risk of stomach, breast, and esophageal cancers. Among nearly 35,000 women in Iowa, those who drank at least two cups a day of tea experienced 60 percent less kidney and bladder cancer and 32 percent less cancer of the esophagus and colon than non–tea drinkers. So there's some pretty solid evidence that catechin-rich tea helps guard against cancer.

Quercetin is among the top flavonoids in our diets, present in fruits, vegetables, and tea. A study published in the March 2001 issue of *Carcinogenesis* reported that quercetin deterred the changes that make prostate cells cancerous and that it may retard the cancer's spread. A 25-year follow-up study involving nearly 10,000 Finnish men showed a reduced risk for lung cancer in cases where the consumption of apples (a major source of quercetin) was high. Quercetin has also been found in animals to inhibit the growth of melanoma, a deadly form of skin cancer.

Scientists believe that quercetin, catechins, and other flavonoids exert their anti-cancer effect by acting as antioxidants. Available from food and internally produced by your body, antioxidants are nutrients that fight free radicals, which are unstable oxygen molecules that attack bodily tissues. Left unchecked, free radicals cause life-shortening diseases, including cancer.

Flavonoids also appear to interfere with the growth and spread of tumors, possibly by inhibiting "tumor angiogenesis." This is an abnormal process by which new blood vessels are formed to feed tumors. When these supply routes are cut off by angiogenesis inhibitors such as flavonoids, tumors can't get the oxygen and nutrients they need to grow. Another way flavonoids fight cancer is by increasing the ability of cells to flush out carcinogens.

All fruits and vegetables are endowed with a variety of cancer-fighting flavonoids. Those highest in catechins and quercetin are listed in the table below. In addition, the counter identifies numerous fruits and vegetables rich in these cancer-protective substances.

ANTI-CANCER FLAVONOIDS

Flavonoid	Major Food Sources
Catechins	Tea (green and black), red wine, chocolate
Quercetin	Onions, apples, black tea, garlic, peppers, berries, grapes, tomatoes

What You Can Do Now

There is no recommended daily intake for flavonoids. However, by eating five or more servings of fruits and vegetables daily (recommended by the American Cancer Society and other groups), you can take in approximately 100 milligrams of flavonoids a day—the amount believed to be the most health-protective. That amount is far greater than the 23 milligrams most people normally consume.

Here are some other ways to sneak more flavonoid-rich foods into your diet:

- Season your foods with chopped garlic or onion.
- Eat a salad every day.
- Eat a variety of fruits and vegetables.
- Try a new fruit or vegetable every week.
- Include at least two vegetables with lunch and dinner.
- Double your portion of vegetables at lunch or dinner.
- Top your breakfast cereal with fresh berries.
- Eat baked potatoes topped with broccoli.
- Add extra vegetables to soups and stews.
- Prepare vegetable or fruit platters to take to parties.
- When eating out, order sandwiches prepared with tomato and lettuce.
- Go meatless several times a week.
- At restaurants, choose vegetarian selections or international dishes.
- Eat vegetable burgers, rather than hamburgers, more frequently.
- For pizza, order one topped with vegetables rather than one with meat.
- Snack on fresh fruits and raw vegetables.
- Start drinking more green or black tea daily to get an extra flavonoid boost.

Carotenoids

Don't risk cancer by shortchanging yourself on orange, red, and yellow fruits and vegetables. They're brimming with carotenoids, a kind of super-antioxidant now making news.

Carotenoids are responsible for the colorful hues of plants and even some animal foods, including salmon and shrimp. But they do more than serve as natural pigments. Carotenoids have "provitamin A activity," meaning that your body produces vitamin A from them, especially beta-carotene (the most well known of the carotenoids).

As antioxidants, these protective nutrients neutralize free radicals at the cellular level, thus protecting cell membranes, DNA, and other cellular components against damage.

The first carotenoid to be isolated was beta-carotene. Today, scientists have discovered more than 600 carotenoids and are reporting that many may be 100 times more powerful than beta-carotene and other antioxidants alone. Among the carotenoids now under the most investigation are alpha-carotene, beta-cryptoxanthin, lutein, lycopene, and zeaxanthin.

Alpha-carotene, which makes up about one-third of the carotenoids in carrots, shows promise in stalling the growth of certain malignant tumors and may be protective against breast cancer. Beta-carotene reduces the risk of cancers of the colon, rectum, breast, uterus, prostate, and lung.

Beta-cryptoxanthin looks promising against breast cancer and lung cancer. Lycopene appears to be protective against cancer of the colon, bladder, and pancreas, but is particularly noteworthy for its role in preventing prostate cancer. In a diet study sponsored by the National Cancer Institute, researchers identified lycopene as being especially powerful against prostate cancer. Tomato sauce, tomatoes, tomato juice, and pizza are the primary sources of lycopene, and those individuals who consumed greater than 10 servings of these combined foods per week had a significantly decreased risk of developing prostate cancer when compared to those who ate less than 1½ servings per week.

Lutein, better known for preventing eye diseases, may guard against cancer of the colon, lung, and breast. Its less-well-known companion carotenoid, zeaxanthin, is linked to a lower risk of breast, cervical, and colon cancers. Both carotenoids are being investigated for their role in preventing skin cancer.

The table below provides an overview of the key carotenoids, their health benefits, and the food sources in which they're found.

CAROTENOIDS

Carotenoid	Health Benefits	Food Sources
Alpha-carotene	Suppresses tumor growth in certain cancers; detoxifies cancer-causing agents.	Carrots, pumpkin, other yellow and orange fruits and vegetables
Beta-carotene	Prevents free radical damage; exerts a protective effect against cancer.	Carrots, pumpkin, other yellow and orange fruits and vegetables
Beta-cryptoxanthin	Prevents damage to cell membranes and to genetic material inside cells.	Oranges, tangerines, peaches, red bell peppers, yellow corn
Lutein	Essential to protect eyes from cataracts and other serious eye problems; shows promise against breast, colon, and lung cancers.	Collard greens, peaches squash, kale, and turnips

Carotenoid	Health Benefits	Food Sources
Lycopene	Lowers risk of developing prostate, lung, pancreatic, bladder, and colon cancers.	Tomatoes, tomato products, guava, watermelon
Zeaxanthin	May play a role in preventing breast, cervical, and colon cancers. Works together with lutein.	Egg yolks, orange peppers

What You Can Do Now

There's no recommended daily requirement for beta-carotene and other carotenoids. However, many health experts recommend six milligrams a day of beta-carotene. When you eat beta-carotene–rich foods, you're automatically getting other carotenoids.

Here are some tips for supercharging your diet with carotenoids:

- Use the counter to identify the best sources of carotenoids. Include these foods in your daily diet.
- Fill your plate with as many colorful vegetables as you can. The more colorful your food selections, the more carotenoids you'll eat.
- Eat canned soups with a tomato base.
- Drink vegetable juices rather than sodas.
- Eat a hefty serving of tomatoes or tomato-based foods at least twice a week.
- Add extra tomato sauce or tomato paste to soups or stews.
- Eat sandwiches and salads with tomatoes.
- Make sure fruits and vegetables are as fresh as possible. Once they're plucked from the vine or

　　harvested from the ground, their antioxidant
　　power starts to dwindle.

- Snack on raw fruits and vegetables to get the most carotenoids. One exception, though, is carrots, which actually release more carotenoids when cooked.
- Enjoy exotic fruits such as guavas or mangoes for a change of pace.
- Blend cooked carrots or pumpkin into a smoothie.

Phytoestrogens

Slowing the rate of growth of prostate and other cancers—even preventing them—may be as simple as eating more soy foods. Soy and other plant foods contain "phytoestrogens," estrogenlike substances. They are also known as isoflavones, and include a subcategory called lignans, which are found in nuts and seeds.

Phytoestrogens act as antioxidants that have been shown to fight free-radical damage that can lead to cancer. These substances also attach themselves to cancer cells and prevent real estrogen from entering the cells and allowing cancer to grow.

Large population studies reveal that men who eat soy are less likely to develop prostate cancer. In fact, soy consumption is proving to be more protective against prostate cancer than any other dietary factor, according to a prostate cancer mortality study conducted in 42 countries. In test tubes, soy protein actually kills off prostate cancer cells.

Where breast cancer is concerned, studies have produced conflicting results. Here's why: Soy contains two phytoestrogens—genistein and diadzein—that exert a number of anticancer activities, according to laboratory studies. Genistein, in particular, has been found to inhibit breast cancer, but not in all cases. In postmenopausal women, who produce little estrogen on their own, genistein may mimic estrogen and actually increase breast cancer risk.

So the jury is still out on the exact role soy plays in preventing breast cancer, or preventing its recurrence. A review study published in 2001 in the *Cancer Journal for Clinicians* could not make a recommendation on soy use for breast cancer survivors, since it had benefits for some but adverse effects for others.

Lignans, however, have been found to lower the incidence of breast and perhaps colon cancer. Lignans are found in numerous plant foods—namely barley, buckwheat, millet, oats, legumes, vegetables, and fruits—but nowhere are they as abundant as in flaxseed. Flaxseed boasts 75 to 800 times more lignans than any other food in the plant kingdom. Unless it is the "high-lignan" variety, however, flaxseed oil contains negligible amounts of lignans, which are nearly all removed during the oil-extraction process.

Foods high in phytoestrogens are listed below. You'll find many others in the counter.

TOP TEN FOOD SOURCES OF PHYTOESTROGENS

Food	Serving Size	Phytoestrogen Content (mg)
Soybeans, cooked from dry	1 cup	220
Soybeans, dry roasted	½ cup	128–167
Nutlettes soy breakfast cereal	½ cup	122
Trail mix, tropical	1 cup	112
Wheat germ oil	1 tbsp.	75
Pistachio nuts, dry roasted	1 oz.	61
Safflower oil	1 oz.	60

Food	Serving Size	Phytoestrogen Content (mg)
Flaxseeds	1 tbsp.	52
Cashews, dry or oil roasted	1 oz.	45
Soy milk (Edensoy Original)	1 cup	41

Source: U.S. Department of Agriculture—Iowa State University, 1999. Database on the isoflavone content of foods.

What You Can Do Now

There is no recommended daily intake for phytoestrogens, although many health authorities recommend 25 to 50 milligrams a day or more. The Food and Drug Administration (FDA) recommends 25 milligrams a day of soy protein, but this recommendation applies only to heart disease, not to cancer, in order to help lower cholesterol.

Here are some suggestions for sneaking more phytoestrogens into your diet:

- Use the counter to select foods highest in phytoestrogens. Some of the best sources are soybeans and soybean products. There is a category in the counter called "Soy Foods and Products" that will help you easily identify high-phytoestrogen foods.
- Use soy milk on your cereal and blended into smoothies.
- Try soy burgers in place of hamburgers.
- Use textured soy protein in recipes calling for ground beef.
- Snack on soy-based nutrition bars rather than on candy bars.
- Use tofu on crackers and rice cakes, and in Italian recipes like lasagna to replace all or part of the ricotta cheese. Tofu can also be blended into shakes and smoothies, plus used as a base for dips.

- Munch on soy nuts or soy chips, available at most health food stores.
- Bake using soy flour to replace some of the flour in recipes.
- Sprinkle flaxseeds on your cereal in the morning—they have a delicious nutty flavor—put them in salads, mix them into yogurt or applesauce, or bake them into muffins and breads in place of nuts.
- Use flaxseeds instead of oil in recipes. Because of their rich oil content, ground seeds can replace all of the oil or shortening in recipes. If a recipe calls for ⅓ cup of oil, for example, use 1 cup of ground seeds instead (a 3 to 1 substitution). Also, 1½ cups of ground flaxseed can replace ½ cup of butter, margarine, or shortening. Baked goods using seeds in this manner will brown more rapidly.

Folate

You probably know it best as folic acid, but folate is the form found in food; folic acid is the supplement form. Folate, a member of the B-complex family of vitamins, is critical for the synthesis, repair, and functioning of DNA, the genetic material of cells.

In fact, numerous scientific experiments have revealed that folic acid deficiencies cause DNA damage that resembles the DNA damage in cancer cells. This finding has led scientists to suggest that cancer could be initiated by DNA damage caused by a deficiency in this B-complex vitamin.

Research shows that folic acid suppresses cell growth in colon cancer. It also prevents the formation of precancerous lesions that could lead to cervical cancer—a discovery that may explain why women who don't eat many vegetables and fruits (good sources of folic acid) have higher rates of this form of cancer. Other studies link low intake of folate to an increased risk of breast, lung, uterine, and pancreatic cancers.

Folate is found in a wide variety of foods—mainly vegetables, cereals, and grains. The table below lists foods highest in folate. Many other high-folate foods are listed in the counter.

TOP TEN SOURCES OF FOLATE

Food	Serving Size	Folate Content (mcg)
Chicken liver, simmered	1 cup	1,078
Total Corn Flakes (General Mills)	1 cup	705
Total (General Mills)	1⅓ cups	676
Total Raisin Bran (General Mills)	¾ cup	675
Kellogg's Product 19 (Kellogg's)	1 cup	672
Chicken giblets, simmered	1 cup	659
Turkey giblets, simmered	1 cup	545
Wheat Chex (General Mills)	1 cup	500
Rice Chex (General Mills)	1 cup	358
Spinach, cooked	1 cup	269

Source: Nutrient Data Laboratory. USDA Nutrient Database for Standard Reference, Release 14. Beltsville, Maryland.

What You Can Do Now

The Daily Reference Intake (DRI) for folate—which refers to the amount of a nutrient you need to prevent chronic disease—is 400 micrograms daily. Here's how you can fortify your diet with more of this vital nutrient:

- Use the counter to identify the richest sources of folate—foods such as cereals, grains, green leafy vegetables, legumes, and lentils, to name just a few.

- Prepare salads using the darkest-leaf lettuce possible (like Romaine). These varieties are higher in folate.
- Look for ways to incorporate spinach and other green leafy vegetables into recipes such as those for soups, lasagna, and casseroles.
- Drink a glass of orange juice most days of the week. It's loaded with folate.
- Switch to folate-fortified cereals.
- Reduce alcohol intake or cut it out altogether. Alcohol blocks the absorption of folate.
- Supplement your diet with commercially prepared liquid nutritional products such as Boost, Ensure, or other meal replacements. These are often fortified with 100 percent of the DRI for folate.
- Consider supplementation with a daily multivitamin/mineral tablet. Your body absorbs only half of the folate you consume, so supplementation is good insurance that you're getting enough. (A caveat: If you're undergoing chemotherapy for cancer, don't take supplements or nutritional beverages containing high levels of folic acid or eat folic acid–fortified foods. Chemotherapeutic agents such as methotrexate interfere with the metabolism of folic acid.)

Selenium

You can get powerful anticancer protection by stocking up on foods rich in selenium, an important antioxidant mineral. Such foods include fish, nuts, and whole grains.

A huge body of evidence proves that diets low in selenium are a significant risk factor for cancers. In studying world populations, scientists have discovered that people with low-selenium diets are more prone to have cancers of the breast, colon, liver, skin, and lung.

Over the years, several studies have suggested that selenium also helps reduce risk of prostate cancer, the second deadliest form of cancer in American men. So intriguing is the selenium/prostate cancer connection that the National Cancer Institute has undertaken a 12-year study involving more than 32,000 men that will explore the role of selenium and vitamin E in preventing prostate cancer.

Selenium works by protecting cells from damage. It may also block the action of carcinogens by interfering with their metabolism.

The table below lists foods high in selenium. You'll find many others in the counter.

TOP TEN FOOD SOURCES OF SELENIUM

Food	Serving Size	Selenium Content (mcg)
Brazil nuts	6–8 nuts (1 oz.)	839
Turkey giblets, simmered	1 cup	321
Chicken liver	1 cup	140
Chicken giblets, simmered	1 cup	136
Clams, cooked	20 clams	122
Mixed nuts, oil roasted with peanuts	1 oz.	118
Tuna, light, canned in water	3 oz.	68
Tuna, light, canned in oil	3 oz.	65
Swordfish	1 piece	64
Tuna salad	5 oz.	58

Source: Nutrient Data Laboratory. USDA Nutrient Database for Standard Reference, Release 14. Beltsville, Maryland.

What You Can Do Now

The DRI for selenium is 55 micrograms daily. To ensure that you're getting ample amounts:

- Use the counter to select high-selenium foods. Some of the best sources include nuts, seeds, fish, whole grains, onions, and broccoli.
- Eat one Brazil nut a day, preferably one that you have unshelled, because it contains around 100 micrograms of selenium (the average selenium supplement contains 50 or 100 micrograms). Grown in the Brazilian jungle where the soil is high in selenium, Brazil nuts are nature's richest source of this important anticancer mineral. Hulled nuts are a good source too, although lower in selenium (12 to 25 micrograms).
- Eat two or three fish meals a week. Fish is packed with selenium. So are meats, but stick to lowfat cuts if you like beef.
- Cook with garlic, another good source of selenium.

Vitamin C

When you think of vitamin C, it's usually in reference to its cold-fighting power. But did you also know that vitamin C—the most commonly supplemented nutrient in the United States—is a potent cancer fighter as well?

That's right. More than a dozen studies have shown that vitamin C, a powerful antioxidant, reduces the risk of almost all forms of cancer, including cancers of the bladder, breast, cervix, colon, esophagus, larynx, lung, mouth, prostate, pancreas, and stomach. Best news of all: Most of the evidence for this anti-cancer benefit comes from studies of high vitamin C intake from foods, not from supplements!

Many researchers believe that vitamin C prevents cancer by disarming free radicals before they can damage DNA and stimulate tumor growth, while others say that the vitamin assists the body's own free radical defense mechanism. Either way, vitamin C is a top cancer fighter.

High vitamin C foods are listed below, and many others can be found in the counter, particularly among fruits and vegetables.

TOP TEN FOOD SOURCES OF VITAMIN C

Food	Serving Size	Vitamin C Content (mg)
Acerola juice	1 cup	3,872
Acerola cherries, raw	1 cup	1,644
Currants, black	1 cup	456
Peppers, sweet, yellow, raw	1 pepper	341
Peaches, frozen, sliced, unsweetened	1 cup	236
Peppers, sweet, red, raw	1 pepper	226
Papaya	1 fruit	188
Guava	1 fruit	165
Chili peppers, green or red, raw	1 pepper	109
Peppers, sweet, green, raw	1 pepper	106

Source: Nutrient Data Laboratory. USDA Nutrient Database for Standard Reference, Release 14. Beltsville, Maryland.

What You Can Do Now

The DRI for vitamin C is 75 milligrams for women and 90 milligrams for men. Female smokers need 110 milligrams a day; male smokers, 130 milligrams a day.

- Use the counter to find high–vitamin C foods. Citrus fruits are excellent choices, as are vegetables such as peppers, cauliflower, tomatoes, and green, leafy vegetables.

- Eat at least one citrus fruit daily. Oranges are an exceptional choice because they contain flavonoids that enhance the absorption of vitamin C.
- Take in extra vitamin C by drinking citrus juice rather than sodas.
- Eat fresh sources of vitamin C whenever possible. Cooking destroys much of the vitamin C in foods.
- Be aware that certain substances inhibit the absorption of vitamin C. These include alcohol, oral contraceptives, smoking, and tetracycline. If using any of these substances, increase your intake of vitamin C–rich foods.

Vitamin E

Skimp on vitamin E in your diet and you may put yourself at risk of developing certain types of cancer. One is breast cancer. A University of California study found that women whose intake of vitamin E from foods was high had a 60 percent lower risk of breast cancer. High vitamin E intake also decreases the risk of cancers of the cervix, colon, mouth, gastrointestinal tract, lungs, and prostate.

However, it's important to add that evidence for an anticancer benefit of vitamin E has been mixed. Some studies show an effect; others do not. Even so, vitamin E's benefit may lie in its synergistic activity with other antioxidants in preventing cancer.

Vitamin E has multiple protective roles in the body. For instance, it helps maintain the integrity of cell membranes, protects against the damaging effects of free radicals, and enhances immunity. It also may block the formation of carcinogens that form in the stomach from nitrites consumed in the diet from smoked and cured meats. Acting as a guardian, vitamin E keeps beta-carotene from being destroyed in the body.

Important food sources of vitamin E include vegetable oils, seeds, nuts, and whole grains. The accompanying chart lists some of the best sources of vitamin E in foods. Many others are listed in the counter.

TOP TEN FOOD SOURCES OF VITAMIN E

Food	Serving Size	Vitamin E Content (IUs)
Total Corn Flakes (General Mills)	1⅓ cup	45
Total Raisin Bran (General Mills)	1 cup	45
Wheat germ oil	1 tbsp.	39
Total cereal (General Mills)	¾ cup	35
Kellogg's Product 19 (Kellogg's)	1 cup	33
Granola, homemade	1 cup	23.5
Trail mix	1 cup	23
Chicken leg, roasted	1 leg	18
Sunflower seeds, dry roasted	1 oz.	12
Almonds	1 oz.	11

Source: Nutrient Data Laboratory. USDA Nutrient Database for Standard Reference, Release 14. Beltsville, Maryland.

What You Can Do Now

The DRI for vitamin E is 22 International Units (IUs) daily. To get more vitamin E in your diet:

- Use the counter to find foods highest in vitamin E. Good sources are cereals, nuts, seeds, vegetable oils, eggs, and green, leafy vegetables.
- Sprinkle nuts and seeds on your salad.
- Add vitamin E–rich wheat germ to cereals, salads, or yogurt.
- Buy cereals fortified with vitamin E.

- Choose "cold-pressed" vegetable oils over refined versions. Oils that have been cold-pressed, which is a processing technique that uses less heat, are higher in vitamin E.
- Avoid regular mega-dosing on vitamin C supplements (1,000 milligrams or more). Excessive doses of vitamin C can interfere with your body's use of vitamin E.

Other Important Cancer-Fighting Agents in Plant Foods

By eating foods rich in nutrients such as vitamin C, vitamin E, folate, and selenium, you are automatically filling up on other nutrients with important disease-fighting properties. They're called "phytochemicals," which means plant chemicals, and they occur naturally in all fruits, vegetables, and grains. Flavonoids, carotenoids, and phytoestrogens are classified as phytochemicals. There are thousands of phytochemicals in foods (one tomato alone contains 10,000), many yet to be identified. They exert their health-protecting action by various biochemical mechanisms, and the results are nothing short of amazing. Phytochemicals appear to protect against not only cancer, but also against heart disease and many other life-threatening illnesses.

In the chart that follows, you will find a list of phytochemicals in foods. With the exception of foods high in flavonoids, carotenoids, and phytoestrogens, most foods have not yet been analyzed for their phytochemical content, which is why these phytochemicals are not listed in the counter. Even so, it's important to know which foods are the best sources of certain phytochemicals so that you can stock your diet with the most protective foods possible.

CANCER-FIGHTING PHYTOCHEMICALS IN PLANT FOODS

Phytochemical	Food Source	Protective Action
Allylic Sulfides	Garlic, onions, and leeks	Ushers carcinogens from the body; decreases tumor reproduction; fortifies the immune system.
Capsaicin	Hot peppers	Neutralizes cancer-causing substances.
Casseic Acid	Fruits	Helps the body produce an enzyme that rids the body of carcinogens.
Catechins	Green and black tea	Appears to be protective against various cancers.
Ellagic Acid	Grapes, nuts	Prevents toxic chemicals from damaging cells; causes cancer cells to kill themselves.
Ferulic Acid	Fruits	Binds to nitrites in foods to prevent them from turning into carcinogenic substances called nitrosamines.
Glucarates	Apples	Helps rid the body of hormones that are linked to breast and prostate cancers.
Indoles	Broccoli, cauliflower cabbage, Brussels sprouts, and kohlrabi	Helps deactivate estrogen, a hormone linked to breast cancer.
Isothiocyanates	Horseradish	Activates an antioxidant enzyme called glutathione, which detoxifies carcinogens.
Limonene	Oranges	Stops damaged cells from uncontrolled growth.
P-coumaric acid and chlorogenic acid	Tomatoes	Prevents the formation of carcinogens called nitrosamines during digestion.

Phytochemical	Food Source	Protective Action
Phenolics	Citrus fruits	Neutralizes carcinogens and stimulates the production of glutathione, a detoxifying enzyme.
Phytates	Grains	Binds to iron, possibly halting the formation of carcinogenic free radicals.
Protease Inhibitors	Legumes	Retards the activity of certain enzymes in cancer cells to slow tumor growth.
Reservatrol	Skin of grapes	Blocks the action of cancer-causing agents; inhibits tumor growth; reverts precancerous cells to normal cells.
Saponins	Onions	Prevents cancer cells from multiplying.
Sulforaphane	Broccoli, cauliflower, cabbage,Brussels sprouts, and kohlrabi	Protects cells against carcinogens.
Triterpenoids	Licorice root	Reduces the risk of breast cancer.

CHAPTER 2

FROM MARKET TO MEALS:

Maximize the Anti-Cancer Power of Your Food

~⌒~

Cancer-conquering, health-building meals begin not only with nutritious food but also with thoughtful food selection and preparation. The juiciest strawberry, the freshest broccoli, the most wholesome rice, or the leanest cut of meat are all for naught if the strawberry isn't refrigerated promptly, the broccoli is overboiled, the rice is rinsed before cooking, or the meat is allowed to char.

Here, then, are vital guidelines, all geared toward healthy food selection, storage, and preparation—guidelines designed to help you harness the maximum cancer-fighting power from your meals. These guidelines work hand in hand with the counter to help you protect yourself against cancer.

Enjoy the Healthy Bounty of Fruits and Vegetables

Nutrients in fruits and vegetables are very sensitive to exposure to heat, light, water, and oxygen. That being the case, you'll want to preserve the nutrient value of your food by following these important tips:

When Shopping

- Look for fresh produce that is crisp and not wilted. Fresh equates with nutritious.
- Avoid buying too much "precut" produce, in which the manufacturer has already diced the vegetables for you and packaged them for convenience. Cutting exposes more surface area to oxygen, which breaks down and destroys nutrients.
- When buying fresh fruits, be on the lookout for bruises on the fruit. Bruising initiates a chemical reaction that causes the nutrient content to dwindle.
- When purchasing a salad mix, look for a colorful medley of greens in the bag. The more color, the more antioxidants, carotenoids, and flavonoids in the salad.
- Always select the brightest, most colorful fruits and vegetables on the shelves. The brighter the color, the more vitamins and other nutrients the produce contains.
- Go for darker shades of green when purchasing lettuce. Dark-leafed vegetables like Romaine lettuce are richer in folate than are lighter green varieties of lettuce such as iceberg.
- Similarly, buy certain vegetables, such as onions and sweet peppers, in all their various colors for a greater array of flavonoids.
- Purchase fresh fruits and vegetables in season when their flavor and nutrition are at peak levels.
- Buy locally grown fresh fruits and vegetables.

They tend to be more nutrient-rich because they come picked right from the field to the produce stand, with less transit time in between. Nutrient loss occurs during the period between harvest and delivery at supermarkets.

- When buying from a salad bar, avoid fruits and vegetables that look brown or slimy. These indicate that the produce has been stored at improper temperatures and may thus be nutritionally bankrupt.

- Berries are highly perishable. At the store, check for freshness by looking at the bottom of the box. Staining indicates that the fruit has been bruised or is overripe, meaning that it will spoil rapidly and that nutrient loss has already set in.

- Look for a bright red color when purchasing strawberries. Bright color signals exceptional nutritional quality. Avoid berries with too much whiteness at the base; they're less nutritious.

- Sniff fruits such as cantaloupe or berries to test for freshness. A pleasant aroma usually indicates good flavor, ripeness, and nutritional goodness. Fruits such as cantaloupes and mangoes should feel somewhat soft to the touch.

- For convenience, don't shun canned foods. Although canning can destroy some vitamin C and B vitamins, canned foods still contain considerable nutrition.

- Buy a variety of fruits and vegetables. The greater the variety of foods you eat, the more health-building nutrients such as vitamins, minerals, phytochemicals, carotenoids, and flavonoids you get in your diet.

Storing Produce

- With the exception of certain fruits like bananas, refrigerate fruits and vegetables promptly. Keeping them cool prevents enzymes from destroying vitamins.

- Eat fresh fruits and vegetables within three to four days of purchase; don't let them sit for too long. The longer produce languishes in your refrigerator, the greater the loss of nutrients. If you can't shop often enough to keep produce fresh, purchase smaller quantities of fruits and vegetables.

  Or, opt for frozen vegetables. They're as high in nutrients as fresh food. Frozen green beans, for example, have more vitamin C than fresh beans stored in the refrigerator for a couple of days. The reason: They were frozen within a few hours of harvesting so, in many cases, their nutritional quality is higher than that of fresh foods. Fresh foods begin to lose nutrients shortly after picking.

Freezing

If you grow your own fruits and vegetables, freezing is a great way to preserve produce, plus lock in nutrition. Here are some pointers:

- Select fruits and vegetables when they're just ripe (but not overripe) and freeze them promptly after harvest. That way, you'll preserve most of their taste and nutrition. The best candidates for freezing are those that you'd normally cook before serving: asparagus, beans, beets, broccoli, Brussels sprouts, carrots, and squash, to name just a few. Among fruits, berries and peaches freeze the best.

- Use freezer-safe containers because they're moisture and vapor proof and thus able to seal out nutrient-destroying air. Freezer bags, wrap, or foil work well too, but make sure you seal these packages as tightly as possible.
- Blanch vegetables prior to freezing them. (Fruits don't need to be blanched.) Blanching inactivates enzymes that break down nutrients. What's more, blanching retains more of the food's vitamin C. The best way to blanch: steam-blanching as opposed to boiling. Steam is gentler on water-soluble nutrients such as B vitamins and vitamin C, and helps preserve nutrient content.
- Eat frozen fruits and vegetables within three to four months. After that period, freezer burn will set in, destroying the food, its flavor, and its nutrient content. B vitamins are particularly vulnerable to lengthy freezing.

Preparing Produce

- Wash fresh produce to remove surface dirt and bacteria, but do not soak it. With soaking, nutrients leach out into the water. Misting, a grocery store process used on certain vegetables, improves humidity to reduce moisture loss from vegetables. It does not affect nutrient loss.
- Eat fruits and vegetables raw whenever possible. Generally, raw produce is healthier. In one interesting study, blood levels of vitamins A and E rose significantly in people who ate raw fruits and vegetables for just one week. One exception to the "raw rule": When cooked, carrots yield more carotenoids.
- Limit cutting and dicing of fruits and vegetables

in order to prevent their surfaces from overexposure to vitamin-destroying oxygen. As an alternative, cut fruits and vegetables into larger pieces and cover them. Serve as close to mealtime as possible.

- Avoid peeling, too. Nutrients and fiber are lost when produce is peeled.
- Don't discard the outer leaves of greens. They contain more nutrients than the inner portions do.
- When boiling, make sure the cooking temperature of the liquid is reached before adding the food. Return the liquid to a boil as quickly as possible after the food has been added.
- Cook foods for the shortest amount of time possible. Use your microwave for quick cooking and for reheating leftovers. Quick cooking methods at high temperatures with the least exposure to water preserve the greatest amount of nutrients. By contrast, vitamins in vegetables are easily destroyed with prolonged exposure to heat, water, and air. Other good quick-cooking methods include steaming, stir-frying, and grilling.
- Cook vegetables using a steam basket that fits into a saucepan. Fill the saucepan with about an inch or two of water. Place vegetables in the basket and cover the saucepan with a tight-fitting lid. Steam vegetables for a few minutes—until they're tender but still crisp—in order to preserve more nutrients.
- In lieu of a steam basket, fill the saucepan with about an inch of water. Add vegetables so that they are piled above the water line. Cook for just a few minutes. The point is to reduce contact with water. Water dissolves water-soluble vitamins such as vitamin C and the B vitamins.

- Avoid thawing frozen fruits and vegetables prior to cooking. As foods thaw, microorganisms once dormant in the food begin to multiply, spoiling the food. It's better to cook frozen food without letting it thaw first.
- With canned food, try to serve its liquid with the food because there are nutrients in the liquid.
- Use any leftover cooking water or canned liquid for soups, sauces, and broths.
- Cook fruits and vegetables with their skins on; this helps lock in nutrients. Consider mashing red potatoes with their skins on for greater nutritional value.
- Never overcook vegetables. It destroys vitamin C, which is highly sensitive to heat. In fact, prolonged boiling robs vegetables of 33 to 90 percent of their vitamin C.
- Minimize reheating of food to reduce further nutrient losses.
- Crush or dice garlic prior to cooking in order to liberate its many beneficial cancer-fighting substances.

Going With the Grain

Grains are less perishable than fruits and vegetables and, under most circumstances, will last indefinitely when properly stored. Even so, grains still require some attention to proper storage and preparation. Here are a few key tips to ensure that you get the most from your grains:

- Choose the most nutritious grains—those that have undergone the least processing. Brown rice, for example, is higher in nutrients and fiber than white rice. That's because white rice has been stripped of its husk, germ, and bran layers during processing. Similarly, rolled oats are generally more nutritious than instant oats.

- Select whole grains—oats, bulgur wheat, rice, and so forth—more often than ready-to-eat cereals. Whole grains tend to be higher in nutrients and fiber than many packaged cereals. Also, bread made from whole grain has several times the fiber found in white bread.
- Store grains in a dark, dry spot in tightly sealed containers. If you live in a humid climate, you can store grains safely in the refrigerator for up to a year.
- Never pre-soak rice or other grains prior to cooking. Pre-soaking washes away nutrients and devitalizes the grain. (It is often recommended that some rices, such as basmati, be pre-soaked; however, this is not always necessary and may result in a mushy texture due to the water that is absorbed.)

Ensuring the Healthiest Meat and Other Proteins

The type of meat you eat and the way you cook it can affect your cancer risk. To minimize that risk:

- Limit your consumption of smoked and nitrite-cured meats. High incidences of esophageal and stomach cancers have been detected in populations who eat large amounts of these foods.
- Grill safely. When the fat from broiling, charring, or grilling foods drips or splatters onto the heat

source, it may be transformed into potentially cancer-causing chemicals, called HAs (heterocyclic amines). These chemicals can then rise from the smoke and deposit onto the cooking food. Smoking and browning of meats will also cause HAs to form.

If the food is charred or otherwise overcooked, HAs can form on the food itself. In fact, a study of women who ate hamburger, steak, and bacon "very well done" showed that they were 4½ times more likely to get breast cancer than those who ate their meats "rare" or "medium."

The moral here: Cut back your use of these cooking methods. Roast, steam, or stew meats instead. These cooking methods keep meat moist, preventing the formation of nasty HAs. Another tip: Marinate meat or poultry prior to grilling it. Marinating slashes HA levels drastically.

- Be careful not to undercook meat, poultry, or fish, however. Undercooking increases the risk that illness-causing bacteria will form on the food. With meat, for example, cook it to the medium rare or medium stage to be on the safe side. Chicken and fish should be fully cooked.
- Opt for veggie or soy burgers. HAs form only in muscle tissue, so meat substitutes, even if grilled, can't fall prey to these cancer-causing substances.

Organic Foods—Are They Healthier?

These days, many people are opting to go "organic." Do you get a health advantage by buying organic foods?

Technically, the term "organic" doesn't describe

how nutritious a food is. Rather, it means that the food has been produced, stored, processed, and packaged without the use of synthetic fertilizers, herbicides, fungicides, or pesticides.

In general, organically grown foods are grown in soil enriched with organic fertilizers and are treated only with nonsynthetic pesticides. Organic farms use a soil-building program that promotes vibrant soil and healthy plants, usually including crop rotations and biological pest control. If a food is organic, its label will say so.

To help you decide whether to go organic, the table below lists the pros and cons of organically grown food.

GOING ORGANIC

Pros	Cons
• May offer higher nutritional content than conventional food, according to some studies.	• May be less fresh. Organic produce may take longer to get to supermarkets than conventional produce does; the slow movement from field to market may cause wilting and nutrient losses.
• Allowed to ripen naturally, which increases nutrient content.	Spoils faster because no preservatives are used.
• Uses natural fertilizers that contain more nutrients (namely zinc and copper) than do most synthetic fertilizers.	• Costs more than its conventional counterparts due to labor-intensive farming methods. Depending on supply and demand, this difference can be quite significant. (Organic food, however, can be inexpensive when purchased in bulk.)
• May reduce health risks associated with pesticides. Organic produce is grown without pesticides or chemical fertilizers; it uses nontoxic natural pesticides instead.	• Lacks the same cosmetic appeal as commercially grown foods due to lack of preservatives and enhancers; organic oranges, for example, tend to look greenish.
• Offers better flavor.	
• Less harmful to the environment.	

CHAPTER 3

THE 10-STEP ANTI-CANCER DIET

~

If you're ready to fine-tune your diet for maximum cancer protection, here's just what you need: the 10-Step Anti-Cancer Diet. Manageable and easy to follow, it's based on recommendations from the American Institute for Cancer Research, the American Cancer Society, and other leading health organizations. In addition to diet, remember that it's vital to get regular exercise, stop smoking, and have regular medical screenings as part of your overall cancer protection program.

Step 1: Slash the Fat.

Adjust your fat intake to roughly 20 percent or less of your total calories and your saturated fat intake to 10 grams a day or less. As an example, let's say you eat around 2,000 calories a day. Four hundred of those calories can come from fat (2,000 x 20% = 400). There are nine calories in each gram of fat, and this means you can eat about 44 grams of total fat daily ($400 \div 9 = 44$). Of that allotment, 10 grams a day or less can come from saturated fat.

Avoid fats designated as "trans-fat," which are synthetic fats found in stick margarine, shortening, fast foods, and many processed foods. Diets overloaded with these may increase your risk of breast cancer.

Don't shun "good fats" either—namely olive oil, canola oil, and peanut oil. Moderate amounts have been found in research to be cancer-protective.

Step 2: Eat Five or More Servings of Fruits and Vegetables Every Day.

Eating a plant-based diet ensures that you get the greatest variety of anti-cancer nutrients. Every day, strive to eat five or more servings of a diverse array of fruits and vegetables. Examples of a serving include one medium piece of fruit, one-half cup of canned fruit, one cup of fruit or vegetable juices, one cup of raw vegetables, or one-half cup of cooked vegetables. Typical serving sizes are also listed in the counter.

An easy way to make sure you get the variety you need is to eat one or more servings a day from each of the following groups:

- Citrus fruits
- Non-citrus fruits, including berries
- Cruciferous vegetables such as broccoli, Brussels sprouts, or cabbage
- Green and dark-green leafy vegetables, including spinach and Romaine lettuce
- Yellow/orange or red vegetables such as sweet peppers, carrots, and squash.

Step 3: Eat Tomatoes and Tomato Products at Least Twice a Week.

Tomatoes deserve a place in the anti-cancer food hall of fame—if there were such a place! That's because they're brimming with lycopene, a powerful cancer-preventing carotenoid. In fact, tomatoes appear to be protective against more cancers than any other vegetable. That being so, make every effort to eat more of them. Each week, try to consume two or more servings of tomatoes or tomato-based products.

(Other lycopene-loaded foods include red grapefruit, watermelon, and guava.)

Step 4: Go with Grains, Legumes, and Root Vegetables Seven or More Times a Day.

Each day, eat seven or more servings of a variety of whole grains and cereals, legumes, and root vegetables. A typical serving is one-half cup cooked whole grain cereal or rice, one slice of bread, one-half cup cooked pasta, one-half cup cooked legumes, or one medium baked potato or sweet potato.

To ensure that you get ample servings of these foods, try to eat one or more servings from these food groups:

- Cereals (brans, wheat, oatmeal, granola bars, high-fiber cereal, or multi-grain cereal)
- Whole grains or whole grain products (barley, brown rice, bulgur wheat, couscous, wild rice, whole grain bread, or pasta)
- Legumes (kidney beans, garbanzo beans, black beans, lima beans, lentils, and others)

- Root vegetables (beets, potatoes, sweet potatoes, yams, and others)

Step 5: Get Your Fiber Fix—
Between 25 and 35 Grams a Day.

The standard advice for fiber intake is to consume between 25 and 35 grams a day. Whole grains, high-fiber cereals, beans and legumes, fruits, vegetables, nuts, and seeds are super sources of fiber that help keep your digestive tract free from cancer-causing substances. If you follow the guidelines in Steps 2 through 4, you should have no trouble obtaining the recommended daily amount of fiber.

Step 6: Enjoy More Soy at Least Once a Day.

Soy foods are supercharged with several anti-cancer substances, including isoflavones, saponins, and protease inhibitors. And because soy foods are protective against several types of cancer and other life-threatening diseases, health experts are now recommending that Americans eat at least 25 grams of soy protein a day, or 25 to 50 milligrams of phytoestrogens (roughly the amount in a traditional diet in Japan, where women seldom get breast cancer).

You can easily get those amounts by eating a cup of cooked soybeans, a cup or two of fortified soy milk, a cup of tofu, or a soy protein shake made with soy protein isolate powder.

Step 7: Dish Out More Fish—
Two to Three Times a Week.

Good-for-you fats called omega-3 fatty acids are abundant in certain types of fish, namely salmon, sardines, mackerel, swordfish, and tuna. Omega-3 fatty acids have been found in studies to reduce the risk of breast cancer. Plus, seafood is packed with cancer-fighting selenium. Try to eat two to three fish meals a week. A typical serving is three to four ounces, about the size of the palm of your hand.

While increasing your fish intake, reduce your consumption of red meat to less than three ounces, no more than a few times a week. Red meat is typically high in fat and, in excess, is considered a risk factor for many cancers.

Step 8: Eat Lowfat Dairy Products
at Least Twice a Day.

With the nutritional spotlight on fruits and vegetables, dairy products don't normally come to mind as cancer-fighters. But they are. Dairy products contain beneficial nutrients that may help you resist cancer, namely calcium, vitamin D, probiotics, and conjugated linoleic acid (CLA). Here's a rundown:

The Calcium-Cancer Connection

Known best as a bone builder, calcium has been shown to cut the risk of colon cancer in half, according to two large health surveys conducted by Harvard researchers. One survey evaluated 626 colon cancer cases among the 88,000 women enrolled in the Nurses Health Study; the other, 399 men with colon cancer who were among the 47,000 people enrolled in the Health Professionals Follow-Up Study. Basically, both surveys discovered that people who consumed between 700 milligrams and 800 milligrams of calcium a day slashed their risk of left-side colon cancer by 40 to 50 percent.

Further, a Columbia University study that looked into the calcium-cancer connection found that that an intake of 1,500 milligrams daily of calcium from low-fat dairy products reduced the rate of abnormal cell growth in the colon, plus caused some precancerous cells to revert to normal.

The DRI for adults for calcium is 1,000 milligrams for men and women, ages 19–50 and 1,200 milligrams for men and women ages 51–70+. You can obtain calcium not only from dairy products but also from broccoli, green leafy vegetables, and calcium-fortified juices.

The Sunlight Vitamin

Vitamin D, a nutrient that helps your body absorb calcium, may lower the risk of breast cancer. This was discovered in research showing that women who had the most sun exposure—our major source of vitamin D—had fewer cases of breast cancer. Sunlight activates a substance in the skin and turns it into vitamin D. All you need is about 5 to 15 minutes of sunlight exposure two to three times a week to get ample vitamin D.

Conveniently too, many milk products, which are great sources of calcium, are routinely fortified with vitamin D. So if you drink milk, you're automatically getting a vitamin D supplement. The DRI for vitamin D is 5 micrograms for men and women ages 19–50, 10 micrograms for men and women ages 51–70, and 15 micrograms for men and women ages 70+.

Probiotics Are Anti-Cancer

Probiotics are healthy bacteria found in yogurt, kefir, buttermilk, and other fermented milk products. Basically, they help maintain the health of the digestive tract, preventing the growth of yeast, salmonella, E. coli, and other nasty germs. The two best-known probiotics are *L. bulgaricus* and *Lactobacilli*. In numerous studies, both have demonstrated anti-tumor activity, particularly against colon cancer. And in at least one study, *Lactobacilli* prevented recurring tumors in bladder cancer patients.

A Fat That Fights Cancer

CLA is a naturally occurring fat present in dairy products (most notably, milk fat), as well as in meat, sunflower oil, and safflower oil. It is formed when the bacteria in a cow's gut breaks down the essential fatty acid, linoleic acid, in the food the animal eats.

CLA's cancer-fighting properties were discovered in a rather serendipitous way. While investigating carcinogens that occur in grilled meats, University of Wisconsin researchers found that CLA blocked the formation of cancer-causing substances. This amazing finding led to more intensive research on CLA's potential as a cancer-fighter. Many animal studies have since found that it suppresses mammary cancer and skin cancer.

Published in 1996, a large-scale study conducted by Finland's National Public Health Institute produced compelling evidence of CLA's anti-cancer benefit in humans. Women who drank milk regularly for 25 years slashed their odds of getting breast cancer by 50 percent, compared to non–milk drinking women. The investigators zeroed in on CLA as the likely agent for the protective effect, since the fatty acid is highly concentrated in milk fat.

A word of important advice: There's no CLA in fat-free milk, so many medical experts are recommending that women switch to 1% lowfat milk (which contains CLA) to get possible protection against breast cancer.

Step 9: Water Your Body.

A little-known fact is that low water intake is a risk factor for certain types of cancer—namely cancers of the urinary tract, colon, and breast. One study found that patients with urinary tract cancer (bladder, prostate, kidney, and testicle) drank significantly smaller quantities of fluid compared with healthy controls.

In another study, researchers discovered that women who drank more than five glasses of water a day had a 45 percent lower risk of colon cancer, compared to those who consumed less than two glasses a day. For men, the risk was cut by 32 percent.

Even more fascinating: A pilot study reported that the odds of developing breast cancer were reduced by 79 percent, on average, among women who drank eight to 10 glasses of water a day.

The reason for water's anti-cancer effect is unclear, but scientists and nutritionists believe that the more fluid you drink, the faster you flush the toxins and carcinogenic substances out of your body.

Try to drink eight to 10 glasses of pure water a day. In addition to water, drink tea—green or black—to the tune of several cups a day. Both types of tea are loaded with cancer-fighting antioxidants.

Step 10: Limit or Avoid Cancer-Causing Substances.

These include cured and smoked meats, which contain known carcinogens called nitrates and nitrites; pickled foods; charred foods; and packaged and highly processed convenience foods, which are chemical- and preservative-laden.

Drinking alcohol is not recommended, either, since alcohol consumption has been associated with breast cancer, liver cancer, and cancers of the head and neck. If you do drink, limit your alcohol intake to less than two drinks daily for men and one for women.

It should be mentioned that there is interest in the role of flavonoids that exist in red wine and in some beers for reducing the risk of certain cancers. At present, the effects of such flavonoids on reducing cancer risk are not known. You can obtain the same beneficial flavonoids from consuming five or more daily servings of fruits and vegetables.

Keeping Track

Using the recommendations explained above, I've created a worksheet to help you keep track of your weekly intake of anti-cancer foods. The worksheet lists the servings of specific groups of foods you need daily or weekly and is organized into one calendar week. Whenever you eat a specific food, simply check off that food in the space provided. This worksheet can serve as a daily reminder of how well you're doing.

Day	Fat	Fruits/Vegetables	Tomato/Tomato Products	Grains, Legumes, Root Vegetables	Fiber	Soy	Fish	Lowfat dairy	Water
	20% of daily calories 10 gm or less saturated fat	5 or more servings daily	2 servings weekly	7 or more servings daily	25–35 gm daily	25 gm daily	2–3 servings a week	2–3 servings daily	8–10 glasses daily
Sun.	☐	Citrus: ☐ Non-citrus: ☐ Brassica: ☐ Green/dark-green leafy: ☐ Yellow/orange or red: ☐	Tomato: ☐	Cereal: ☐☐ Whole grains: ☐☐ Legumes: ☐☐ Root Vegetables ☐☐	☐	☐	☐☐	☐☐☐	☐☐☐ ☐☐☐
Mon.	☐	Citrus: ☐ Non-Citrus: ☐ Brassica: ☐ Green/dark-green leafy: ☐ Yellow/orange or red: ☐	Tomato:	Cereal: ☐ Whole grains: ☐ Legumes: ☐ Root vegetables: ☐☐	☐	☐	☐☐☐	☐☐☐	☐☐☐ ☐☐☐
Tues.	☐	Citrus: ☐ Non-citrus: ☐ Brassica: ☐ Green/dark-green leafy: ☐ Yellow/orange or red: ☐	Tomato:	Cereal: ☐ Whole grains: ☐ Legumes: ☐☐☐ Root vegetables: ☐☐	☐	☐	☐☐☐	☐☐☐	☐☐☐ ☐☐☐

Wed. ☐

Citrus: ☐
Non-citrus: ☐
Brassica: ☐
Green/dark-green leafy: ☐
Yellow/orange or red: ☐

Tomato: ☐

Cereal: ☐☐
Whole grains: ☐☐
Legumes: ☐☐
Root vegetables: ☐☐

☐   ☐   ☐   ☐   ☐☐☐ ☐☐☐

Thurs. ☐

Citrus: ☐
Non-citrus: ☐
Brassica: ☐
Green/dark-green leafy: ☐
Yellow/orange or red: ☐

Tomato: ☐

Cereal: ☐☐
Whole grains: ☐
Legumes: ☐☐
Root vegetables: ☐☐

☐   ☐   ☐   ☐☐☐ ☐☐☐

Fri. ☐

Citrus: ☐
Non-citrus: ☐
Brassica: ☐
Green/dark-green leafy: ☐
Yellow/orange or red: ☐

Tomato: ☐

Cereal: ☐☐
Whole grains: ☐☐
Legumes: ☐
Root vegetables: ☐☐

☐   ☐   ☐   ☐☐☐ ☐☐☐

Sat. ☐

Citrus: ☐
Non-citrus: ☐
Brassica: ☐
Green/dark-green leafy: ☐
Yellow/orange or red: ☐

Tomato: ☐

Cereal: ☐☐
Whole grains: ☐☐
Legumes: ☐☐
Root vegetables: ☐

☐   ☐   ☐   ☐☐☐ ☐☐☐

CHAPTER 4

A SAMPLE ANTI-CANCER MENU*

~

The three-day menu below illustrates what an ideal anti-cancer diet looks like in real life. Recipes follow the sample menu plan.

Day 1

BREAKFAST
Phyto-Fit Fruity Shake
1 slice whole wheat bread, toasted
1 cup green tea

MID-MORNING SNACK
1 cup freshly squeezed carrot juice

*The nutrients in this menu and these recipes were figured using Nutribase Clinical software, which does not calculate carotenoids or flavonoids, even though this menu and its recipes are naturally high in these nutrients.

LUNCH
Mexican Bean Stew
Broccoli Carrot Salad
1 small piece cornbread
1 cup 1% milk

MID-AFTERNOON SNACK
1 nonfat granola/raisin bar (Health Valley)
1 cup nonfat lemon yogurt

DINNER
Marinated Salmon with Papaya Salsa
1 medium sweet potato
½ cup Brussels sprouts
Tomato slice

Nutrition information for Day 1: 1,834 calories; 36 grams of fat; 6 grams of saturated fat; 39 grams of fiber; 22 milligrams of phytoestrogens; 261 micrograms of folate; 80 micrograms of selenium; 236 milligrams of vitamin C; and 6 IUs of vitamin E.

Day 2

BREAKFAST
Blueberry Brancakes
2 tbsp. light blueberry syrup
½ cup blueberries
1 cup green tea

MID-MORNING SNACK
1 cup vegetable juice
2 nonfat rice cakes

LUNCH
Mediterranean Salad with High-Lignan Flaxseed Oil Dressing
1 cup cooked brown rice
1 cup soy milk
Pumpkin Delight

MID-AFTERNOON SNACK
Tasty Trail Mix (¼ cup)
1 cup nonfat cherry yogurt

DINNER
Super-Stuffed Red Peppers
½ cup mashed butternut squash
½ cup cooked spinach
1 cup watermelon balls

Nutrition information for Day 2: 1,828 calories; 46 grams of fat; 4 grams of saturated fat; 42 grams of fiber; 30 milligrams of phytoestrogens; 322 micrograms of folate; 180 micrograms of selenium; 578 milligrams of vitamin C; and 11 IUs of vitamin E.

Day 3

BREAKFAST
1 cup cooked oatmeal with 2 tbsp. wheat bran
1 cup fortified soy milk
1 cup Concord grape juice
1 cup green tea

MID-MORNING SNACK
1 cup acerola cherry juice
1 whole grain bagel

LUNCH
   Veggie burger (Green Giant Harvest Burger) on whole-grain bun
   Coleslaw (1 cup shredded cabbage with 2 tbsp. Hidden Valley nonfat coleslaw dressing)
   1 cup sliced beets, cooked

MID-AFTERNOON SNACK
   1 lowfat energy bar
   1 cup nonfat vanilla yogurt

DINNER
   Zucchini Lasagna
   1 whole wheat dinner roll
   Tropical Salad

Nutrition information for Day 3: 1,771 calories; 42 grams of fat; 9 grams of saturated fat; 39 grams of fiber; 15 milligrams of phytoestrogens; 1,000 micrograms of folate; 44 micrograms of selenium; 4 grams of vitamin C; and 57 IUs of vitamin E.

Recipes

PHYTO-FIT FRUITY SHAKE

½ cup silken tofu
1 cup calcium-fortified orange juice
1 tbsp. wheat bran
½ cup crushed pineapple (canned in its own juice, drained)
½ frozen banana
1 tbsp. honey
½ tsp. coconut extract

Place all ingredients in a blender and blend until smooth. Makes 1 large serving.

Nutrition information per serving: 249 calories; 4.6 grams of fat; 0.6 gram of saturated fat; 9 grams of fiber; 9.5 milligrams of phytoestrogens; 17 micrograms of folate; 1 microgram of selenium; 5 milligrams of vitamin C; and 0.5 IUs of vitamin E.

MEXICAN BEAN STEW

2 tbsp. olive oil
1 tbsp. chopped garlic
1 onion, chopped
1 green pepper, chopped
2 15-oz. cans kidney beans, drained
1 15-oz. can corn, drained
1 4-oz. can green chilies
2 28-oz. cans crushed tomatoes
1 packet taco seasoning mix

In a large saucepan, sauté garlic, onion, and green pepper in olive oil until tender. Add rest of ingredients and bring to a simmer. With lid on, simmer for 20 minutes. Makes 4 servings.

Nutrition information per serving: 330 calories; 6.3 grams of fat; .01 gram of saturated fat; 13 grams of fiber; 5 milligrams of phytoestrogens; 8 micrograms of folate; 0.4 micrograms of selenium; 54 milligrams of vitamin C; and 0.25 IUs of vitamin E.

BROCCOLI CARROT SALAD

6 cups broccoli florets
1 4-oz. jar pimentos, drained
½ cup chopped red onions
1 cup carrots, grated
½ cup shredded soy cheddar cheese

Dressing:
1 cup fat-free mayonnaise (Kraft)
2 tbsp. seasoned rice vinegar
1 tsp. salt
2 tsp. sugar
1 tsp. garlic powder

Combine vegetables and cheese. Mix well. Mix together all ingredients for dressing. Blend with a whisk until smooth. Pour dressing over vegetable and cheese mixture, and mix well. Refrigerate for at least 4 hours. Makes 6 servings.

Nutrition information per serving: 95 calories; 0.35 grams of fat; 0.05 gram of saturated fat; 1 gram of fiber; 4 milligrams of phytoestrogens; 56 micrograms of folate; 2.4 micrograms of selenium; 85 milligrams of vitamin C; and 2 IUs of vitamin E.

MARINATED SALMON WITH PAPAYA SALSA

4 pieces of salmon fillet (about 4 oz. each)
1 cup teriyaki sauce
1 tbsp. ground ginger

Marinate the salmon in the teriyaki sauce with ginger for 30 minutes. Grill salmon over medium heat until fish flakes easily with a fork. Serve with Papaya Salsa (see page 60). Makes 4 servings.

Papaya Salsa

2 cups cubed fresh papaya
1 medium red onion, chopped
1 medium fresh jalapeño pepper, chopped
4 tbsp. cilantro
1 tsp. salt
2 tsp. canola oil
2 tsp. apple cider vinegar

Mix all ingredients and serve over grilled salmon. Makes 4 servings.

Nutrition information per serving: 321 calories; 15 grams of fat; 2.7 grams of saturated fat; 3 grams of fiber; 4 milligrams of phytoestrogens; 66 micrograms of folate; 42 micrograms of selenium; 57 milligrams of vitamin C; and 2 IUs of vitamin E.

BLUEBERRY BRANCAKES

1 egg
½ cup All-Bran with Extra Fiber
1 cup 1% milk
½ cup self-rising flour
½ cup whole wheat flour
1 tbsp. brown sugar
1 tbsp. canola oil
1 tsp. baking powder
½ cup fresh blueberries
2 tbsp. wheat bran

Beat egg until fluffy. Let All Bran soak in milk until soft. Add flours, sugar, canola oil, baking powder, and All Bran and milk mixture to egg. Blend until smooth. Stir in blueberries.

Heat stick-free griddle. For each pancake, pour about 3 tablespoons of batter onto griddle. Cook pancakes until puffy and dry around edges. Before flipping, sprinkle each pancake with some of the bran. Turn and cook the other side until brown. Makes 8 pancakes (2 pancakes per serving).

Nutrition information per serving: 215 calories; 5 grams of fat; 0.3 grams of saturated fat; 7.5 grams of fiber; 0 milligrams of phytoestrogens; 57 micrograms of folate; 9 micrograms of selenium; 7 milligrams of vitamin C; and 1.7 IUs of vitamin E.

MEDITERRANEAN SALAD

½ cup garbanzo beans
2 oz. feta cheese
½ onion, chopped
½ cup cooked string beans
½ yellow pepper, chopped
1 cup Romaine lettuce, shredded

Arrange beans, cheese, onion, string beans, and yellow pepper on a bed of Romaine lettuce. Drizzle with 1 tbsp. of High-Lignan Flaxseed Oil dressing. Makes 1 serving.

Nutrition information per serving: 306 calories; 13 grams of fat; 8.5 grams of saturated fat; 10 grams of fiber; 8 milligrams of phytoestrogens; 53 micrograms of folate; 9 micrograms of selenium; 194 milligrams of vitamin C; and 0.14 IU of vitamin E.

High-Lignan Flaxseed Oil Dressing

¼ cup white balsamic vinegar
3 tbsp. water
1 package (0.75 ounce) Good Seasonings Garlic &
*   Herb salad dressing mix*
½ cup high-lignan flaxseed oil

Place vinegar and water in a container with a tight-fitting lid. Add salad dressing mix and shake vigorously until well blended. Add oil and shake again until well blended. Makes 16 1-tbsp. servings. Can be refrigerated for up to four weeks.

Nutrition information per serving: 66 calories; 7 grams of fat; 0.6 grams of saturated fat; 0 grams of fiber; phytoestrogens—not available; 0 micrograms of folate; 0 micrograms of selenium; 0 milligrams of vitamin C; and 0 IUs of vitamin E.

PUMPKIN DELIGHT

1¾ cups of cold 1% milk
1 package Jell-O Fat-Free Sugar-Free Instant Pudding Mix (1.5 oz.)
1 15-oz. can pumpkin
½ tsp. cinnamon
¼ tsp. ginger
⅛ tsp. ground cloves

Place milk in a bowl. Add remaining ingredients and mix with a wire whisk until smooth. Pour into small cups or custard bowls and refrigerate for at least 3 hours. Makes 4 servings.

Nutrition information per serving: 115 calories; 1.3 grams of fat; 0.2 gram of saturated fat; 3.2 grams of fiber; 0 milligrams of phytoestrogens; 13 micrograms of folate; 0.43 microgram of selenium; 5 milligrams of vitamin C; and 1.7 IUs of vitamin E.

TASTY TRAIL MIX

6 Brazil nuts, whole hulled nuts cut into halves
½ cup dried Mission figs, diced
½ cup dried apricots, diced
½ cup walnuts
¼ cup sunflower seeds (dry roasted kernels)

Mix all ingredients. Store in refrigerator. Makes 6 ¼-cup servings.

Nutrition information per serving: 190 calories; 12 grams of fat; 1.6 grams of saturated fat; 5 grams of fiber; 0 milligrams of phytoestrogens; 15 micrograms of folate; 145 micrograms of selenium; 0.5 milligram of vitamin C; and 5 IUs of vitamin E.

SUPER-STUFFED RED PEPPERS

6 red sweet bell peppers
1 lb. ground chicken
1 medium onion, chopped
2 medium tomatoes, chopped
½ cup chopped pecans
1 cup chopped shiitake mushrooms
1 cup cooked bulgur wheat
1 tbsp. fresh basil, chopped
⅛ tsp. red pepper
1 tsp. salt
¼ tsp. black pepper

Cut out tops of red peppers and remove seed core. Boil peppers in a large saucepan of water until just tender. Drain on a paper towel.

Brown chicken; drain any fat. Add onion, tomatoes, pecans, mushrooms, wheat, and spices. Sauté until all vegetables are soft. Stuff peppers with mixture and bake at 350° F. for 25 minutes. Makes 6 servings.

Nutrition information per serving: 294 calories; 13 grams of fat; 0.85 gram of saturated fat; 5 grams of fiber; 18 milligrams of phytoestrogens; 40 micrograms of folate; 20 micrograms of selenium; 275 milligrams of vitamin C; and 0.15 IU of vitamin E.

ZUCCHINI LASAGNA

6 medium zucchini, sliced lengthwise into strips
2 tbsp. water
1 lb. bulk turkey sausage
1 medium onion, chopped
1 tbsp. chopped garlic
1 tbsp. brown sugar
3 tbsp. fresh basil, chopped
2 tbsp. fresh oregano, chopped
6 sprigs of fresh rosemary, chopped (leaves only)
1 tsp. salt
1 28-oz. can crushed tomatoes
1 small can (6 oz.) tomato paste
1 cup ricotta cheese
1 cup tofu, soft silken
½ cup reduced-fat Parmesan cheese
2 cups soy mozzarella cheese, shredded

Cook and stir sausage, onion, and garlic in a large skillet until sausage is brown; drain. Stir in herbs and brown sugar, tomatoes, and tomato paste. Bring to a boil, then let simmer covered for 30 minutes.

Place half of zucchini slices in a microwave dish with a tablespoon of water. Cover dish with plastic wrap, turning back one corner to vent. Microwave on high for 6 minutes or until zucchini is just tender. Let cooked zucchini drain on a paper towel; pat dry to remove excess moisture. Repeat with remainder of zucchini.

Mix ricotta cheese, tofu, and Parmesan cheese in a small bowl.

Spread a thin layer of the meat sauce in an ungreased rectangular baking dish. Top with several zucchini slices. Spread ½ of cheese/tofu mixture over zucchini; spread with another thin layer of meat sauce. Sprinkle with ⅔ cup soy mozzarella cheese. Repeat layering process with zucchini, remaining cheese/tofu mixture, sauce, and ⅔ cup soy mozzarella cheese. Top with any remaining zucchini slices and sprinkle with remaining soy mozzarella cheese.

Bake uncovered in 350° oven for 45 minutes. Remove from oven and let stand for 15 minutes. Makes 8 servings.

Nutrition information per serving: 437 calories; 22 grams of fat; 7 grams of saturated fat; 4 grams of fiber; 2 milligrams of phytoestrogens; 40 micrograms of folate; 9 micrograms of selenium; 28 milligrams of vitamin C; and 0.5 IU of vitamin E.

TROPICAL SALAD

2 ripe mangoes, peeled and diced
1 banana, sliced
1 cup chopped orange sections
1 cup fresh pineapple, diced

Mix fruits and serve immediately. Makes 6 ½-cup servings.

Nutrition information per serving: 90 calories; 0.4 gram of fat; 0.09 gram of saturated fat; 3 grams of fiber; 5 milligrams of phytoestrogens; 25 micrograms of folate; 1 microgram of selenium; 41 milligrams of vitamin C; and 1.4 IUs of vitamin E.

CHAPTER 5

THE ANTI-CANCER NUTRITION COUNTER

⌒

FOODS THAT COMBAT CANCER is the only compilation you'll find of cancer-fighting substances found in everyday foods. It contains data on calories, fat, saturated fat, fiber, flavonoids, carotenoids, phytoestrogens, folate, selenium, vitamin C, and vitamin E for basic foods, brand-name foods, health foods, and fast foods—all right at your fingertips.

How to Locate Foods

Foods are alphabetized in food categories as well as under individual categories so that you'll have no trouble finding whatever you want to look up. If you're looking for a particular food, look for it alphabetically under its category. Let's say, for example, you're looking for carrots. Check the table of contents, where you'll find an alphabetized listing of food categories, and go to "vegetables and legumes." Turn to the page where the vegetable listings begin and go to the Cs.

Vegetables are listed in alphabetical order, so it's easy to locate *carrots.* Under *carrots,* you'll find information for various types of carrots, including raw, canned, frozen, and cooked from fresh. That way, you'll be able to compare the nutrient content of different preparations quickly and easily.

Among the categories in the counter are *dinners* and *entrées.* Dinners represent entire meals, and they generally include an entrée such as fish or chicken, a side vegetable, and a dessert. Entrées, on the other hand, refer to only the principal food in a meal, such as baked chicken or lasagna.

The fast food category is arranged for ease of use as well. Under fast foods, foods are categorized alphabetically into breakfast foods, burgers, desserts, Mexican foods, sandwiches, pasta, pizza, poultry, and so forth. You can look at each of these categories and compare the nutrient quality of a Burger King selection to a Hardee's selection, for example.

In the interest of good health, certain foods have been excluded from the counter, namely highly processed foods and those high in fat or sugar. Even though you'll find foods like cakes, ice cream, puddings, fast foods, and hot dogs in the counter, in most cases only their lowfat and/or reduced-sugar counterparts have been included.

How to Identify Anti-Cancer Nutrients

Each food entry lists the following information in this order: food name, serving size, caloric content, and the amount of each of the following (in grams, milligrams, micrograms, or other relevant measurement): total fat, saturated fat, fiber, flavonoids, carotenoids, phytoestrogens (PE), folate, selenium, vitamin C, and vitamin E. Here's a closer look:

Serving Size

Serving size refers to the standard amount of food suggested by the U.S. Department of Agriculture and the food industry.

Calories

This describes the amount of energy provided by one serving, and can be used to help you accurately plan your meals if you're following a weight-reducing diet. Generally, most people can lose weight safely by following a diet that supplies 1,200 to 1,500 calories a day.

Fat

Much research strongly suggests that dietary fat (mainly saturated fat and trans-fats) plays a role in causing cancer, particularly breast and prostate cancers. In the counter, fat content per serving is presented as total fat/saturated fat. For example: for one cup of brown rice (instant), the entry is 2 grams/0 grams.

Your daily fat intake should be 20 percent or less of your total calories. On a 2,000-calorie-a-day diet, that translates into 44 grams of fat. This calculation is determined in the following manner: 2,000 calories x 20% = 400 ÷ 9 (number of calories in a gram of fat) = 44. Of your daily fat portion, 10 grams a day or less can come from saturated fat.

Look for foods lowest in saturated fat. Generally, you'll find such foods under fruits, vegetables, cereals, grains, soy foods, fish, poultry (white meat), and other lowfat entries.

Keep in mind that there are good fats that protect against cancer. These include olive oil and oils found in fish.

Fiber

Hundreds of studies support the cancer-fighting power of fiber. To harness its protective benefit, the National Research Council recommends 20 to 35 grams of fiber a day. In the counter, fiber content is presented in grams (gm). Your best fiber bets are found in cereals, grains, flours, fruits, certain dinners and entrées, nuts and seeds, vegetables, and some vegetarian-type fast foods. Look for foods that contain at least 2.5 to 3 grams of fiber per serving.

Flavonoids

Flavonoids are near-miracle workers when it comes to cancer prevention. You'll find these amazing nutrients mostly in fruits, fruit juices, vegetables, and vegetable juices, as well as in beverages such as coffee, tea, wine, and some beers.

Although there is no official recommended dietary intake for flavonoids, health experts advise consuming 100 milligrams a day. You can easily obtain this amount by eating five or more servings of fruits and vegetables a day.

The flavonoid content of foods has not been as extensively measured as other anti-cancer nutrient content has been. But where flavonoid content is available, the counter provides the amount in milligrams (mg).

Carotenoids

Found abundantly in fruits and vegetables, carotenoids shore up a powerful defense against cancer. Foods particularly high in carotenoids include those found in the following categories: beverages/fruit juices, beverages/vegetable juices, fruits, tomatoes and tomato products, and vegetables.

Recommended intakes have not yet been established for carotenoids, although health experts advise 6 milligrams a day for beta-carotene. By eating a variety of brightly colored fruits and vegetables each day, you'll obtain an ample array of carotenoids from your diet.

The counter provides the amount of carotenoids in foods, designated either by micrograms (mcg) or milligrams (mg), and identifies specific carotenoids as follows: alpha-carotene (AC), beta-carotene (BC), beta-cryptoxanthin (BCR), lutein and zeaxanthin (LU+Z), and lycopene (LYC).

Phytoestrogens

You'll find phytoestrogens mostly in vegetables, especially soy and soy products, as well as in other plant-based foods such as nuts and seeds. Phytoestrogens have been found in research to fight various forms of cancer, including cancers of the breast, prostate, and colon.

There is no recommended intake for phytoestrogens. However, health experts advise eating 25 to 50 milligrams a day of these cancer-fighting agents. In the counter, specific phytoestrogens are identified as follows: daidzen (D), genistein (G), daidzen and genistein (D/G), or lignans (L). A designation without D, G, D/G, or L means that analysis of that food for specific phytoestrogens is lacking. Phytoestrogens are measured in either micrograms (mcg) or milligrams (mg).

Folate

Folate is an important anti-cancer nutrient because deficiencies of this vitamin have been associated with an increased risk of breast, colon, lung, uterine, and pancreatic cancers. In the counter, look for high-folate foods among cereals, diet and sports products, flours, grains, some milk beverages, pasta, vegetables, and some meats. Folate is measured in micrograms (mcg). The Daily Reference Intake (DRI) for folate is 400 micrograms.

Selenium

This antioxidant mineral helps reduce the risk of prostate, lung, and colon cancers. You'll find it mostly in cereals, eggs, fish, grains, meats (beef, ham, lamb, pork, and poultry), nuts, seeds, and vegetables. Certain bread products such as bagels are also high in selenium. In the counter, the amount of selenium in foods is presented in micrograms (mcg). The DRI for selenium is 55 micrograms.

Vitamin C

A growing number of studies reveal that vitamin C, a powerful antioxidant, is effective in lowering the risk of developing cancer of the bladder, breast, cervix, colon, esophagus, lung, mouth, prostate, stomach, and throat. In the counter, you'll find vitamin C primarily in fruits, fruit juices and punches, and vegetables and vegetable juices. Many foods are enriched with vitamin C as well, including cereals and diet and sports products. There is also considerable vitamin C in some fast foods and soups. The amount of vitamin C per serving appears in milligrams (mg). The DRI for vitamin C is as follows: 75 milligrams (women); 90 mil-

ligrams (men); 110 milligrams (women who smoke);
and 130 milligrams (men who smoke).

Vitamin E

This vitally important antioxidant is protective
against a number of cancers, and you'll find it in cereals, grains, soy foods, nuts, seeds, vegetable oils, and
vitamin E–enriched foods. The amount of vitamin E
per serving appears in International Units (IUs). The
DRI for vitamin E is 22 IUs.

Top Sources of Anti-Cancer Nutrients

Wherever a nutrient amount appears in bold type,
this indicates that the serving supplies 25 percent or
more of the recommended daily intake for that particular nutrient and is therefore considered a high source.

Abbreviations and Symbols

As you locate the foods in which you're interested,
keep in mind the following abbreviations and symbols:

Measurements:
fl. oz.	fluid ounce
gm	gram
IUs	International Units
mcg	microgram
mg	milligram
oz.	ounce
tbsp.	tablespoon
tsp.	teaspoon
t	trace
w/	with
w/o	without

Food Descriptions and Nutrients

0	zero (no nutrient value)
AC	alpha-carotene
BC	beta-carotene
BCR	beta-cryptoxanthin
D	daidzen
D/G	daidzen and genistein
G	genistein
L	lignan
LU+Z	lutein and zeaxanthin
LYC	lycopene
na	information not available *(Note: A designation of "na" does not mean an absence of a particular nutrient, only that analysis of that food for that nutrient is lacking.)*
PE	phytoestrogens
Vit. C	vitamin C
Vit. E	vitamin E

All the information in the Anti-Cancer Nutrition Counter is based on information from the United States government, from producers of brand-name foods, and from fast-food restaurant chains. Also consulted were two important databases, the U.S. Department of Agriculture (USDA)-Iowa State University Database on the Isoflavone Content of Foods and the USDA-Nutrition Coordinating Center (NCC) Carotenoid Database for U.S. Foods; numerous journal articles that analyzed nutrient content of various foods; and various computer- and Web-based sources, including Diet Expert, Foodcount.com, and Nutribase.

This counter provides you with information to help

you make the best possible food choices and take steps toward preventing cancer. Take it wherever you go—to the grocery store, restaurants, and so forth—to make sure that you're eating right and eating well.

Food	Serving Size	Calories	Fat/Sat. Fat (gm)	Fiber (gm)	Flavonoids (mg)	Carotenoids (mcg or mg)	PE (mcg or mg)	Folate (mcg)	Selenium (mcg)	Vit. C (mg)	Vit. E (IUs)
BEEF											
Brisket, braised*	3 oz.	185	8.6/3	0	0	0	0	7	21	0	0.2
Chuck roast, baked*	3 oz.	250	16/6	0	0	0	0	8.5	21	0	0.25
Chipped, dried	1 slice	15	0.4/.1	0	0	0	0	1	5.6	0	0
Corn beef, canned	1 slice	52.5	3/1.3	0	0	0	0	2	9	0	0.05
Eye of round*	3 oz.	165	7/2.6	0	0	0	0	6	22	0	0.2
Flank steak*	3 oz.	176	8.6/3.7	0	0	0	0	7	20.5	0	0
Hamburger:											
Beef patty, cooked from frozen	3 oz. (1 patty)	240	17/6.5	0	0	0	0	7.6	18	0	0
Extra lean, broiled medium	3 oz.	218	14/5.5	0	0	0	0	7.6	16	0	0.23
Extra lean, broiled well done	3 oz.	225	13.4/5	0	0	0	0	9	19	0	0.23
Lean, broiled medium	3 oz.	231	16/6	0	0	0	0	7.6	24.6	0	0.26
Lean, broiled well done	3 oz.	238	15/6	0	0	0	0	9	21.5	0	0.26
Regular, broiled medium	3 oz.	246	17.5/7	0	0	0	0	7.6	16	0	0.3
Regular, broiled well done	3 oz.	248	16.5/6.5	0	0	0	0	8.5	18	0	0.3
Porterhouse steak, broiled*	3 oz.	253	19/7	0	0	0	0	6	19	0	0.26
Rib-eye steak, broiled	3 oz.	188	10/3.7	0	0	0	0	6.7	20	0	0.2
Round tip, roasted*	3 oz.	186	9.6/3.6	0	0	0	0	7	23	0	0.2
T-bone steak, broiled*	3 oz.	238	16.5/6.4	0	0	0	0	6	19	0	0.24
Sirloin steak, broiled*	3 oz.	211	12/5	0	0	0	0	7.6	25	0	0.23
Tenderloin, roasted*	3 oz.	239	16/6	0	0	0	0	5	20.5	0	0

*trimmed to ⅛" fat, all grades

75

Food	Serving Size	Calories	Fat/Sat. Fat (gm)	Fiber (gm)	Flavonoids (mg)	Carotenoids (mcg or mg)	PE (mcg or mg)	Folate (mcg)	Selenium (mcg)	Vit. C (mg)	Vit. E (IUs)
Variety meats:											
Brain, pan-fried	3 oz.	167	13.5/3	0	0	0	0	5	22	3	0
Heart, simmered	3 oz.	149	5/1.4	0	0	0	0	1.7	33	1.3	0.9
Liver, pan-fried	3 oz.	185	7/2.3	0	0	0	0	187	48.5	19.5	0.9
Tongue, baked	3 oz.	237	17/7.5	0	0	0	0	4	14	.3	0.5
BEVERAGES/ALCOHOLIC/BEER											
Beer, light	12 fl. oz.	99	0/0	0	na	0	t (D/G)	14.5	4.2	0	0
Beer, nonalcoholic	12 fl. oz.	70	0/0	0	na	0	na	na	na	na	0
Beer, regular	12 fl. oz.	146	0/0	0.7	177–358	0	t (D/G)	21	4.3	0	0
BEVERAGES/ALCOHOLIC/DISTILLED LIQUORS											
80 proof	1 fl. oz.	64	0/0	0	t–9	0	na	0	0	0	0
90 proof	1 fl. oz.	73	0/0	0	t–9	0	na	0	0	0	0
100 proof	1 fl. oz.	82	0/0	0	t–9	0	na	0	0	0	0
BEVERAGES/ALCOHOLIC/WINE											
Champagne	1 wine glass (3.5 fl. oz.)	72	0/0	0	na	0	na	1.1	0.2	0	0
Dessert, dry	1 wine glass (3.5 fl. oz.)	130	0/0	0	na	0	na	0.4	0.4	0	0
Dessert, sweet	1 wine glass (3.5 fl. oz.)	158	0/0	0	na	0	na	0.4	0.5	0	0

Food	Serving Size	Calories	Fat/Sat. Fat (gm)	Fiber (gm)	Flavonoids (mg)	Carotenoids (mcg or mg)	PE (mcg or mg)	Folate (mcg)	Selenium (mcg)	Vit. C (mg)	Vit. E (IUs)
Nonalcoholic	1 wine glass (3.5 fl. oz.)	6	0/0	0	na	0	na	0.3	0.1	0	0
Red	1 wine glass (3.5 fl. oz.)	74	0/0	0	**28–81**	0	na	2.06	0.2	0	0
Rosé	1 wine glass (3.5 fl. oz.)	73	0/0	0	**28–81**	0	na	1.13	0.2	0	0
Sherry	1 wine glass (3.5 fl. oz.)	158	0/0	0	na	0	na	0.4	0.5	0	0
White	1 wine glass (3.5 fl. oz.)	70	0/0	0	**1**	0	na	0.2	0.2	0	0
Wine cooler	1 drink (7 fl. oz.)	105	0/0	.1	na	1.8 mcg (BC)	na	2.5	0.3	3.8	0
BEVERAGES/COFFEE											
Brewed, decaf	1 cup	4.7	0/0	0	na	0	na	0	0.23	0	0
Brewed, regular	1 cup	4.7	0/0	0	**177**	0	na	0.2	0.23	0	0
Prepared from instant, decaf	1 cup	3.5	0/0	0	na	0	na	0	0.18	0	0
Prepared from instant, regular	1 cup	3.6	0/0	0	na	0	na	0	0.18	0	0
BEVERAGES/FRUIT JUICES											
Acerola juice	1 cup	56	0.7/0.16	0.7	na	740 mcg (BC)	na	34	0.2	**3,872**	0.15

77

Food	Serving Size	Calories	Fat/Sat. Fat (gm)	Fiber (gm)	Flavonoids (mg)	Carotenoids (mcg or mg)	PE (mcg or mg)	Folate (mcg)	Selenium (mcg)	Vit. C (mg)	Vit E (IUs)
Apple juice, canned, unsweetened, w/ added Vit. C	1 cup	117	0.27/0.04	0.25	0.6	0	na	0.25	0.24	103	0.05
Apple juice, canned, unsweetened, w/o added Vit. C	1 cup	117	0.27/0.05	0.25	0.6	0	na	0.25	0.24	2.2	0.05
Apple juice, from concentrate, diluted, unsweetened, w/ added Vit. C	1 cup	112	0.24/0.04	0.24	0.6	0	na	0.7	0.24	60	na
Apple juice, from concentrate, diluted, unsweetened, w/o added Vit. C	1 cup	112	0.24/0.04	0.24	0.6	0	na	0.7	0.24	1.4	na
Apricot nectar, w/ added Vit. C	1 cup	140.5	0.23/0.01	1.5	na	2 mg (BC)	na	3.3	0.5	137	0.3
Apricot nectar w/o added Vit. C	1 cup	140.5	0.23/0.01	1.5	na	2 mg(BC)	na	3.3	0.5	1.5	0.3
Grape juice, from concentrate, diluted, sweetened, w/ added Vit. C	1 cup	127.5	0.23/0.07	0.25	1.15	15 mcg (BC)	na	3.25	0.25	60	0.2
Grape juice, unsweetened, w/ added Vit. C	1 cup	152	0.2/0.1	0.25	1.15	15 mcg (BC)	na	6.5	0.25	60	0
Grape juice, unsweetened, w/o added Vit. C	1 cup	154	0.2/0.06	0.25	1.15	15 mcg (BC)	na	6.6	0.25	0.25	0
Grapefruit juice, pink, fresh	1 cup	93	0.25/0.03	na	46–199	15 mcg (BC)	na	25	na	94	na

78

Food	Serving Size	Calories	Fat/Sat. Fat (gm)	Fiber (gm)	Flavonoids (mg)	Carotenoids (mcg or mg)	PE (mcg or mg)	Folate (mcg)	Selenium (mcg)	Vit. C (mg)	Vit. E (IUs)
Grapefruit juice, white, fresh	1 cup	96	0.25/0.03	0.25	46–199	15 mcg (BC)	na	25	0.25	94	0.2
Grapefruit juice, sweetened, canned	1 cup	115	0.22/0.03	0.25	46–199	na	na	26	0.25	67	0.2
Grapefruit juice, unsweetened, canned	1 cup	94	0.25/0.03	0.25	46–199	15 mcg (BC)	na	26	0.25	72	0.2
Grapefruit juice, from concentrate, diluted, sweetened	1 cup	118	0.25/t	0.25	46–199	12 mcg (BC)	na	9	0.25	81.5	0.2
Grapefruit juice, from concentrate, diluted, unsweetened	1 cup	101	0.32/0.05	0.25	46–199	13 mcg (BC)	na	9	0.25	83	0.2
Lemon juice, bottled	1 tbsp.	3.2	0.04/t	0.06	t	1.8 mcg (BC)	na	1.5	0.01	3.8	0.02
Lemon juice, from 1 lemon	1 fruit	12	0/0	0.19	t	7 mcg (BC)	na	6	0.05	22	0.06
Lime juice, bottled	1 tbsp.	3.2	0.04/t	0.06	na	1.8 mcg (BC)	na	1.5	t	4	t
Lime juice, from 1 lime	1 fruit	10		0.2	na	2 mcg (BC)	na	3	t	11	t
Mango nectar, canned	1 cup	146	0.3/0.1	1.8	na	1.7 mg (BC)	na	7	0.7	19	2
Orange juice, fresh	1 cup	112	0.5/0.06	0.5	52	298 mcg (BC)	na	75	0.25	124	0.3
Orange juice, canned, unsweetened	1 cup	105	0.35/0.04	0.5	52	269 mcg (BC)	na	45	0.25	86	0.3
Orange juice, from carton, unsweetened	1 cup	109.5	0.7/0.07	0.5	52	269 mcg (BC)	na	45	0.25	82	na

Food	Serving Size	Calories	Fat/Sat. Fat (gm)	Fiber (gm)	Flavonoids (mg)	Carotenoids (mcg or mg)	PE (mcg or mg)	Folate (mcg)	Selenium (mcg)	Vit. C (mg)	Vit. E (IUs)
Orange juice, from concentrate, diluted	1 cup	112	0.15/0.01	0.5	52	119 mcg (BC)	na	109	0.25	97	0.75
Orange-grapefruit juice, canned, unsweetened	1 cup	106	0.25/0.03	0.25	na	178 mcg (BC)	na	35	0.25	72	0.25
Papaya nectar, canned	1 cup	142.5	0.4/0.1	1.5	na	165 mcg (BC)	na	5	0.75	7.5	0.08
Peach nectar, canned, w/ added Vit. C	1 cup	134	0.05/t	1.5	na	388 mcg (BC)	na	3.5	0.5	67	t
Peach nectar, canned, w/o added Vit. C	1 cup	134	0.05/t	1.5	na	388 mcg (BC)	na	3.5	0.5	13	t
Pineapple juice, canned, unsweetened, w/ added Vit. C	1 cup	140	0.2/0.01	0.5	na	0	na	58	0.25	60	0.08
Pineapple juice, canned, unsweetened, w/o added Vit. C	1 cup	140	0.2/0.01	0.5	na	0	na	58	0.25	27	0.08
Pineapple juice, from concentrate, unsweetened, diluted	1 cup	130	0.07/t	0.5	na	0	na	26.5	0.25	30	0.03
Pineapple-grapefruit juice, bottled, canned, or carton	1 cup	117.5	0.2/0	0.4	na	8 mcg (BC)	na	42	0.3	50	0.15
Pineapple-orange juice, canned	1 cup	123	0/0	0.25	na	135 mcg (BC)	na	27	0	56	0

Food	Serving Size	Calories	Fat/Sat. Fat (gm)	Fiber (gm)	Flavonoids (mg)	Carotenoids (mcg or mg)	PE (mcg or mg)	Folate (mcg)	Selenium (mcg)	Vit. C (mg)	Vit. E (IUs)
Pineapple-orange-banana juice, carton	1 cup	127	0.2/0	0.8	na	68 mcg (BC)	na	65	0.4	**60**	0.5
Prune juice, bottled or canned	1 cup	182	0.07/t	2.6	na	0	na	1	1.5	10.5	0.03
Strawberry/banana-orange juice, from carton	1 cup	126	0.7/0.2	2.6	na	28 mcg (BC)	na	37	0.2	**20**	0.5

BEVERAGES/JUICE DRINKS & PUNCHES

Food	Serving Size	Calories	Fat/Sat. Fat (gm)	Fiber (gm)	Flavonoids (mg)	Carotenoids (mcg or mg)	PE (mcg or mg)	Folate (mcg)	Selenium (mcg)	Vit. C (mg)	Vit. E (IUs)
Cranberry apple drink, bottled	1 cup	165	0/0	0.24	na	0	na	0.5	0	**78**	0
Cranberry grape drink, bottled	1 cup	137	0.25/0.08	0.24	na	28 mcg (BC)	na	1.7	0	**78**	na
Cranberry juice cocktail, bottled	1 cup	144	0.25/0.02	0.25	na	0	na	0.5	0	**89.5**	0
Cranberry juice cocktail, low-calorie, bottled	1 cup	45	0/0	0	na	0	na	0.5	0	**76**	0
Fruit punch drink, made from frozen, or canned (Hawaiian Punch, Hi-C)	1 cup	116	0/0	0.2	na	15 mcg (BC)	na	3.2	0	**73**	0
Grape juice drink, canned	1 cup	125	0/0	0.25	na	0	na	2	0	**40**	0
Kool-Aid, with sugar, prepared, w/ added Vit. C	1 cup	88	0/0	0	na	1.2 mcg (BC)	na	0.2	0.1	**28**	0

Food	Serving Size	Calories	Fat/Sat. Fat (gm)	Fiber (gm)	Flavonoids (mg)	Carotenoids (mcg or mg)	PE (mcg or mg)	Folate (mcg)	Selenium (mcg)	Vit. C (mg)	Vit. E (IUs)
Kool-Aid, low-calorie, prepared, w/ added Vit. C	1 cup	43	0/0	0	na	14 mcg (BC)	na	5	0	77.5	0
Lemonade, from concentrate, diluted	1 cup	99	0/0	0	na	33 mcg (BC)	na	5	0	10	na
Limeade, from concentrate, diluted	1 cup	101	0/0	0.25	na	0	na	2.5	0	7	na
Tang Instant Breakfast Juice Drink, prepared with water, w/ Vit. C added	1 cup	119	0/0	0	na	0	na	0	0.2	74	4
Splash, all flavors (Campbell's)	1 cup	267	0.1/0	0.7	na	3 mg (BC)	na	2.4	0.7	61	0
Splash, diet, all flavors (Campbell's)	1 cup	19	0/0	0	na	na	na	na	na	78	9
Sports drinks:											
Gatorade (Quaker Oats)	1 cup	60	0/0	0	na	0	na	0	0.7	0	0
Gatorade Light (Quaker Oats)	1 cup	26	0/0	0	na	0	na	0	0.2	15	0
BEVERAGES/VEGETABLE JUICES											
Carrot juice, canned	1 cup	94	0.35/0.06	1.8	na	3.6 mg (BC)	na	9	1.4	20	0.03
Tomato juice	1 cup	41	0.15/0.02	1	12	816 mcg–1 mg (BC) 149 mcg (LU+Z) 23 mg (LYC)	na	48	1.2	44.5	3.3

Food	Serving Size	Calories	Fat/Sat. Fat (gm)	Fiber (gm)	Flavonoids (mg)	Carotenoids (mcg or mg)	PE (mcg or mg)	Folate (mcg)	Selenium (mcg)	Vit. C (mg)	Vit. E (IUs)
Tomato juice, low sodium	1 cup	41	0.15/0.02	2	na	816 mcg–1 mg (BC) 23 mg (LYC)	na	48	1.2	44.5	3.3
Tomato juice, with clam juice	1 cup	35	0.2/0.1	0.7	na	610 mcg (BC)	na	37	1.3	33	2.5
Vegetable juice with tomato	1 cup	46	0.2/0.03	2	na	520 mcg (AC) 1.7 mg – 2 mg (BC) 198 mcg (LU+Z) 24 mg (LYC)	na	51	1.2	67	1
BEVERAGES/NON-MILK, GRAIN BASED											
Cereal grain beverage (Kaffree Roma)	1 cup	6	0/0	0	na	na	na	na	na	na	na
Rice beverage, canned (Rice Dream)	1 cup	120	2/0.2	0	na	na	na	na	na	1.2	2.6
Rice beverage original (Rice Dream)	1 cup	120	2/0	0	na	na	na	na	na	0	na
Rice beverage w/ soy (Eden Foods)	1 cup	120	3/0.5	0	na	na	na	na	na	na	na
BEVERAGES/TEA											
Green tea, brewed	1 cup	2.4	0/0	0	230	0	0.12 mg	12.3	0	0	0
Herbal tea, brewed	1 cup	2.3	0/0	0	na	0	na	1.4	0	0	0
Iced tea, with lemon (Nestlé)	1 cup	88	0.7/0.05	0	na	na	na	na	na	na	na

83

Food	Serving Size	Calories	Fat/Sat. Fat (gm)	Fiber (gm)	Flavonoids (mg)	Carotenoids (mcg or mg)	PE (mcg or mg)	Folate (mcg)	Selenium (mcg)	Vit. C (mg)	Vit. E (IUs)
Tea (black), brewed	1 cup	2.4	0/0	0	163	0	na	12.3	0	0	0
Tea, instant, sweetened, w/ added Vit. C	1 cup	88	0/0	0	na	0	na	9.6	0.26	23	na
BREADS, MUFFINS, AND ROLLS											
Bagels:											
Blueberry, refrigerated (Lenders)	1 bagel	209	1.3/0.3	2	t	t	na	60	na	0	na
Cinnamon raisin	1 bagel, 3" dia.	156	1/0.15	1.3	0	0	na	51	18	0.4	0.13
Egg	1 bagel, 3" dia.	158	1.2/0.2	1.3	0	na	na	50	17.4	0.34	na
Multigrain	1 bagel, 3" dia.	148	0.7/0.1	4	0	t	na	51	18	0	0.45
Oat bran	1 bagel, 3" dia.	145	0.7/0.1	2	0	0	na	46	19.5	0.11	0.11
Plain, enriched	1 bagel, 3" dia.	157	1/0.12	1.3	0	0	na	50	18	0	0.03
Whole wheat	1 bagel, 3" dia.	151	0.8/0.1	5.3	0	0	na	34	30	0	0.75
Biscuits:											
From home recipe	1 biscuit 2¼" dia.	212	9.8/2.6	0.9	0	0	18 mg	37	12	0.12	1.17

Food	Serving Size	Calories	Fat/Sat. Fat (gm)	Fiber (gm)	Flavonoids (mg)	Carotenoids (mcg or mg)	PE (mcg or mg)	Folate (mcg)	Selenium (mcg)	Vit. C (mg)	Vit. E (IUs)
From mix	1 biscuit, 3" dia.	191	7/1.6	1	0	0	na	30	3.5	0.23	na
From refrigerated dough	1 biscuit, 2¼" dia.	95	4/1	0.5	0	0	na	17	6	0	0.8
From refrigerated dough, lowfat	1 biscuit, 2" dia.	59	1/0.25	0.37	0	0	na	19.5	4.3	0	0.2
Bread crumbs	½ cup	395	5.4/2.3	2.4	0	0	na	109	10.7	0	0.86
Bread sticks	1 stick, 7⅞" x ⅝"	41	1/0.14	0.3	0	0	na	12	3.75	0	0.22
Bread stuffing	½ cup	178	8.6/1.7	3	0	0	na	101	50	0	2
Bread stuffing, cornbread	½ cup	179	9/1.8	3	0	52 mcg (BC)	na	97	31	0.8	2
Breads:											
Boston brown, canned	1 slice	88	0.7/0.13	2	0	na	na	5	10	0	0.38
Branola	1 slice	89	1.2/0.3	1.4	0	0	na	25	11	0	0.3
Cinnamon	1 slice	69	0.9/0.1	0.6	0	0	na	25	7	0	0.15
Cracked wheat	1 slice	65	1/0.23	1.4	0	0	na	15	6.3	0	0.22
Egg	1 slice	115	2.4/0.3	1	0	0	2.8 mg	42	12	0	0.36
French or Vienna	1 medium slice	68.5	0.75/0.16	0.75	0	0	na	24	7.9	0	0.1
Fruit and nut	1 slice	217	10/2	1	t	8.4 mcg (BC)	na	24	8	1.3	1.65
Garlic	1 medium slice	96	3.8/0.7	0.8	na	31 mcg (BC)	na	24	8	0.1	0.75

85

Food	Serving Size	Calories	Fat/Sat. Fat (gm)	Fiber (gm)	Flavonoids (mg)	Carotenoids (mcg or mg)	PE (mcg or mg)	Folate (mcg)	Selenium (mcg)	Vit. C (mg)	Vit. E (IUs)
Granola	1 slice	89	1.2/0.3	1.4	0	0	na	25	11	0	0.3
High fiber, reduced calorie	1 slice	60	0.7/0.2	3	0	0	na	28	6	0.1	0.15
High protein	1 slice	64	0.6/0.1	0.8	0	0	na	27	8.6	0	0
Italian	1 medium slice	54	0.7/0.17	0.5	0	0	na	19	5.4	0	0.1
Low gluten	1 slice	73	1.4/0.2	1.5	0	0	na	19.5	8.6	0	0.3
Mixed grain (7-grain, whole grain)	1 slice	65	1/0.2	1.7	0	0	na	21	7.7	0.08	0.26
Mixed grain, reduced calorie	1 slice	52.5	0.6/0.1	3	0	0	na	19.5	9	0	0
Oat bran	1 slice	71	1.3/0.2	1.3	0	0	na	24	9	0	0.3
Oat bran, reduced calorie	1 slice	46	0.7/0.1	2.7	0	0	na	15	5	0	0.1
Oatmeal	1 slice	72	1.2/0.4	1	0	0	na	17	6.6	0	0.25
Oatmeal, reduced calorie	1 slice	48	0.8/0.14	na	0	0	na	13	5	0.05	0
Pita, white, enriched	1 large, 6.5" dia.	165	0.72/0.1	1.3	0	0	na	57	16	0	0.03
Pita, whole wheat	1 large, 6.5" dia.	170	1.7/0.3	5	0	0	na	22	28	0	0.9
Potato	1 slice	69	0.9/0.1	0.6	0	0	na	25	7	0	0.15
Pumpernickel	1 slice	50	0.6/0.08	1.3	0	0	na	16	5	0	0.13
Pumpernickel, marbled with rye	1 slice	66	0.8/0.1	1.6	0	0	na	22	7	0	0.15
Raisin	1 slice	71	1.1/0.3	1	na	0	na	23	5	0.1	0.3

86

Food	Serving Size	Calories	Fat/Sat. Fat (gm)	Fiber (gm)	Flavonoids (mg)	Carotenoids (mcg or mg)	PE (mcg or mg)	Folate (mcg)	Selenium (mcg)	Vit. C (mg)	Vit. E (IUs)
Rice bran	1 slice	66	1.2/0.5	1.3	0	0	na	17.5	7.8	0	0.34
Rye, light or dark	1 slice	52	0.6/0.12	1.2	0	0	na	17	6	0.08	0.1
Rye, reduced calorie	1 slice	46	0.6/0.08	3	0	0	na	11	6	0.09	0.06
Rye, snack-sized	1 slice	18	0.23/0.04	0.4	0	0	na	6	2	0.03	0.04
Sprouted grain, inc.											
Ezekiel bread	1 slice	65	1/0.2	1	0	0	na	19	8	0	0.15
Sweet potato	1 slice	74	1.6/0.3	0.5	na	190 mcg (BC)	na	23	5.6	0.9	0.3
Sunflower seed	1 slice	75	1.4/0.4	0.5	na	2 mcg (BC)	na	21	7	0.1	0.3
Triticale	1 slice	63	1/0.2	1.6	na	0	na	17	8	0	0.3
Wheat, including											
wheatberry	1 slice	65	1/0.2	1	0	0	na	19	8	0	0.2
Wheat, reduced calorie	1 slice	45	0.5/0.07	2.8	0	0	na	16	7	0.02	0.04
Wheat germ	1 slice	73	0.8/0.2	0.6	0	0	na	26	8	0.06	0.04
White	1 slice	69	0.9/0.1	0.6	0	0	na	25	7	0	0.15
White, prepared from recipe, with 2% milk	1 slice	120	2.4/0.5	0.8	0	0	na	38	9	0.04	0.5
White, reduced calorie	1 slice	48	0.6/0.12	2.2	0	0	na	22	5	0.12	0.05
Whole wheat	1 slice	69	1.2/0.25	2	0	0	na	14	10	0	0.36
Whole wheat, prepared from recipe	1 slice	128	2.5/0.36	2.8	0	0	na	28	18	0	0.6
Cornbread:											
Prepared from home recipe, with 2% milk	1 piece	188	6/1.6	1.4	0	38 mcg (BC)	na	33	6	0.06	na

87

Food	Serving Size	Calories	Fat/Sat. Fat (gm)	Fiber (gm)	Flavonoids (mg)	Carotenoids (mcg or mg)	PE (mcg or mg)	Folate (mcg)	Selenium (mcg)	Vit. C (mg)	Vit. E (IUs)
Prepared from mix	1 piece	140	4.5/1.5	2	0	20 mcg (BC)	na	23	3.6	0.2	0.9
Croissant	1 medium	231	12/6.6	1.5	0	46 mcg (BC)	na	35	13	0.1	0.3
Croutons, plain	½ cup	61	1/0.23	0.75	0	0	na	20	5.5	0	na
English muffins:											
Mixed grain	1 muffin	155	1/1.5	2	0	0	na	53	17	0	0.3
Plain, enriched	1 muffin	134	1/1.5	1.5	0	0	na	46	11.5	0	0.15
Raisin	1 muffin	138.5	1.5/0.23	1.7	0	0	na	46	9	0.17	0.35
Wheat	1 muffin	127	1/0.16	2.6	0	0	na	31	16.7	0	0.4
Whole wheat	1 muffin	134	1.4/0.2	4.4	0	0	na	32	26	0	0.7
Muffins, commercially prepared:											
Blueberry	1 muffin	158	3.7/0.8	1.5	0	10 mcg (BC)	na	26	6	0.6	0.9
Bran	1 muffin	168	5/0.8	4.4	na	0	na	18	11	0	1
Carrot	1 muffin	174	6.6/0.9	1	na	1.4 mg (BC)	na	25	9	0.9	2
Cheese	1 muffin	177	7/2	0.7	0	13 mcg (BC)	na	29	11	0.1	0.7
Corn	1 muffin	160.5	5/1.4	1.2	0	0	na	28.5	7.6	0.05	na
Oat bran	1 muffin	154	4/0.6	2.6	0	0	na	30	6	0	1
Oatmeal	1 muffin	136	3.5/0.9	0.8	0	2.4 mcg (BC)	na	27	10.5	0.1	0.6
Plain	1 muffin	175	6/1.5	0.7	0	3 mcg (BC)	na	32	11.5	0.2	1
Pumpkin	1 muffin	178	4/0.7	1	na	1.9 mg (BC)	na	18	6.6	0.7	1.4
Toaster muffin	1 muffin	110	3.3/0.5	0.6	na	1.8 mg (BC)	na	15.5	6	0	0.5
Zucchini	1 muffin	215	11/1.5	0.8	na	26 mcg (BC)	na	23	8	1	3
Muffins, from home recipe:											
Blueberry	1 muffin	162	6/1	na	t	10 mcg (BC)	na	27	5	0.8	na

88

Food	Serving Size	Calories	Fat/Sat. Fat (gm)	Fiber (gm)	Flavonoids (mg)	Carotenoids (mcg or mg)	PE (mcg or mg)	Folate (mcg)	Selenium (mcg)	Vit. C (mg)	Vit. E (IUs)
Bran	1 muffin	168	5/0.8	4.4	na	0	na	18	11	0	1
Corn	1 muffin	180	7/1.3	na	0	na	na	35	7.6	0.17	na
Plain	1 muffin	169	6.5/1.3	1.5	0	na	na	29	5	0.17	na
Muffins, toaster:											
Blueberry	1 muffin	103	3/0.5	0.6	na	na	na	18	6	0	0.9
Corn	1 muffin	114	4/0.5	0.5	na	na	na	19	5	na	na
Wheat bran	1 muffin	106	3/0.5	3	na	na	na	11.5	7	0	1
Rolls and buns:											
Cloverleaf	1 roll	103	1.8/0.4	1	0	0	na	46	9.5	0	1
Dinner roll, egg	1 roll, 2½" dia.	107.5	2/0.5	1.3	0	0	na	37	10	0	0.38
Dinner roll, plain	1 roll	85	2/0.5	0.9	0	0	na	27	8	0.03	0.38
Dinner roll, rye	1 small, 2⅜" dia.	81	1/0.17	1.4	0	0	na	24	8	0	0.15
Dinner roll, wheat	1 roll	77	1.8/0.4	1	0	0	na	14.5	9	0	0.4
Dinner roll, whole wheat	1 roll, 2½" dia.	96	1.7/0.3	2.7	0	0	na	11	18	0	0.7
French roll	1 roll	105	1.6/0.36	1	0	0	na	36	10.6	0	0.25
Hamburger bun, mixed grain	1 bun	113	2.6/0.6	1.6	0	0	na	41	14	0	0.37
Hamburger bun, plain	1 bun	123	2/0.5	1	0	0	na	41	11	0.04	1
Hard roll, Kaiser	1 roll, 3½" dia.	167	2.5/0.3	1.3	0	0	na	54	22	0	0.3
Hotdog bun, mixed grain	1 bun	113	2.6/0.6	1.6	0	0	na	41	14	0	0.37
Hotdog bun, plain	1 bun	123	2/0.5	1	0	0	na	41	11	0.04	1

89

Food	Serving Size	Calories	Fat/Sat. Fat (gm)	Fiber (gm)	Flavonoids (mg)	Carotenoids (mcg or mg)	PE (mcg or mg)	Folate (mcg)	Selenium (mcg)	Vit. C (mg)	Vit. E (IUs)
Submarine/hoagie bun	1 bun, 8" long	269	5/1	2.5	0	0	na	119	25	0.1	2.3
Tacos:											
Corn, large	1 taco, 6½" dia.	98	4.7/0.7	1.6	0	0	na	22	2.5	0	0.9
Corn, medium	1 taco, 5" dia.	62	3/0.4	1	0	0	na	14	1.6	0	0.6
Flour, large	1 taco, 10" dia.	286	15/3.6	2	0	0	na	46	13.5	0	3.6
Flour, regular	1 taco, 7" dia.	173.5	9/2.2	1	0	0	na	28	8	0	2.2
Tortillas:											
Corn, large	1 tortilla, 8" dia.	73	0.8/0.1	1.7	0	0	na	37.6	2	0	0.15
Corn, medium	1 tortilla, 6" dia.	42	0.5/0.1	1	0	0	na	22	1	0	0
Flour, large	1 tortilla, 10" dia.	218	5/1.2	2	0	0	na	82	16	0	1.2
Flour, medium	1 tortilla, 8" dia.	140	3/0.8	1.4	0	0	na	53	10	0	0.75
Whole wheat, large	1 tortilla, 8" dia.	109	0.7/0.1	3	0	0	na	12.5	28	0	0.9
Whole wheat, medium	1 tortilla, 7" dia.	84	0.5/0.1	2	0	0	na	9.6	22	0	0.75

CAKES, LOWFAT

Food	Serving Size	Calories	Fat/Sat. Fat (gm)	Fiber (gm)	Flavonoids (mg)	Carotenoids (mcg or mg)	PE (mcg or mg)	Folate (mcg)	Selenium (mcg)	Vit. C (mg)	Vit. E (IUs)
Apple Raisin Spice Cake (Weight Watchers)	1 serving	173	4/0.9	1.6	0	70 mcg (BC)	0	21	8	1.5	0.6
Brownie, fudge, nonfat (Entenmann's)	1 piece	110	0/0	1	0	0	0	na	na	0	na
Brownie, peanut butter fudge (Weight Watchers)	1 serving	110	2.5/0.5	3	0	0	0	na	na	0	na
Carrot cake, fat-free (Entenmann's)	1 slice	170	0/0	1	na	na	0	na	na	0	na
Chocolate cake, sugar-free (Sweet 'n' Low)	⅙ cake	150	3/1	1	0	0	0	na	na	0	na
Coffee cake, fruit-topping, fat-free	1 piece	94	0.2/0	0.6	0	1.2 mcg (BC)	0	23	6	0.5	0
Crumb cake, lowfat (Hostess)	1 serving	90	0.5/0	0	0	0	0	na	na	0	na
Cupcake, chocolate, w/frosting, lowfat	1 cupcake	131	1.6/0.5	2	0	0	0	6.5	1.6	0	na
Devil's Food Cake, reduced fat (Sweet Rewards)	1 serving	160	1.5/0.5	1	0	0	0	24	na	0	na
Double Fudge Cake (Weight Watchers)	1 serving	190	4.5/1	2	0	0	0	na	na	0	na
Fudge Iced Chocolate cake, nonfat (Entenmann's)	1 slice	210	0/0	2	0	0	0	na	na	0	na

Food	Serving Size	Calories	Fat/Sat. Fat (gm)	Fiber (gm)	Flavonoids (mg)	Carotenoids (mcg or mg)	PE (mcg or mg)	Folate (mcg)	Selenium (mcg)	Vit. C (mg)	Vit. E (IUs)
German Chocolate Cake (Weight Watchers)	2½-oz. serving	200	7/1	0	0	0	0	na	na	na	na
Lemon cake, w/icing, lowfat (Duncan Hines Delights)	1 piece	382	10/2	0.3	0	44 mcg (BC)	0	26	4	0.1	2
Pineapple cake, fat-free	1 piece	69	0.1/0	0.4	0	0.6 mcg (BC)	0	9	4.5	0.3	0
Pound cake, fat-free	1 slice	79	0.3/0.1	0.3	0	0	0	10	1.5	0	0
Pound cake, chocolate, fat-free	1 slice	77	0.3/0.1	0.6	0	0	0	10	2.4	0.1	0
Pound cake, reduced fat	1 slice	86	2/0.4	0.3	0	0	0	10	4	0.1	0.75
Shortcake Snack (Weight Watchers)	1 serving	170	2/1	0	0	0	0	na	na	na	na
White cake, eggless, lowfat	1 piece	165	3.6/0.6	0.4	0	1.2 mcg (BC)	0	18	6	0.1	1
CEREALS/COLD CEREALS											
100% Bran (Post)	⅓ cup	83	0.6/0.08	8.3	0	0	na	100	na	0	na
100% Natural Oats & Honey (Quaker)	½ cup	213	8/3.5	3.6	0	0	na	12	8	0.15	0.8
40% Bran Flakes (Ralston)	1 cup	159	0.7/0	7	0	0	na	173	na	26	na
All-Bran Bran Buds (Kellogg's)	⅓ cup	83	0.7/0.12	12	0	0	na	90	8.7	15	0.7
All-Bran (Kellogg's)	½ cup	79	0.9/0.2	9.7	0	0	na	90	3	15	0.8

Food	Serving Size	Calories	Fat/Sat. Fat (gm)	Fiber (gm)	Flavonoids (mg)	Carotenoids (mcg or mg)	PE (mcg or mg)	Folate (mcg)	Selenium (mcg)	Vit. C (mg)	Vit. E (IUs)
All-Bran w/ extra fiber (Kellogg's)	½ cup	53	1/0.17	13	0	0	na	120	3	17	1
Almond Delight	½ cup	100	1.5/0.4	1.5	0	56 mcg (BC)	na	92	1	14	0.2
Alpen	½ cup	199	1.8/0.3	5	0	0	na	17	10	5	0.3
Amaranth Flakes	1 cup	134	4/0.8	3.6	0	20 mcg (BC)	na	4	27	1	5
Apple Raisin Crisps (Kellogg's)	1 cup	185	0.5/0.1	4	na	0	na	110	5	0	0.7
Banana Nut Crunch (Post)	1 cup	249	6/0.8	4	0	0	na	100	na	0.12	na
Basic 4 (General Mills)	1 cup	200	3/0.4	3.4	0	0	na	99	9.4	15	1
Bran Chex (Kellogg's)	1 cup	156	1.4/0.2	8	0	0	na	173	4.4	26	0.9
Bran Flakes Kellogg's	¾ cup	95	0.6/0.12	4.6	0	0	na	102	3	15	8
Branola	½ cup	233	5.6/0.9	4.7	0	6.6 mcg (BC)	na	16.5	9.5	0.1	2
Cheerios multigrain (General Mills)	1 cup	112	1/0.25	2	0	0	na	376	5	15	0.3
Common Sense Oat Bran Flakes (Kellogg's)	¾ cup	109	1/0.36	4	0	0	na	90	5	0	0.5
Corn Bran (Quaker)	1 cup	120	1/0.3	6.4	0	30 mcg (BC)	na	134	4	0	0.3
Corn Chex (Ralston)	1 cup	113	0.36/0.07	0.5	0	0	na	336	3	6	0.15
Corn Flakes	1 cup	102	0.2/0.05	0.8	0	0	na	99	1.4	14	0.05
Cracklin Oat Bran (Kellogg's)	¾ cup	225	7/3	6.5	0	0	na	153	12	17	0.55
Crispex (Kellogg's)	1 cup	108	0.3/0.09	0.6	0	0	na	87	3	15	0.18
Crunchy Bran (Ralston)	¾ cup	90	0.9/0.2	5	0	0	na	100	3	3	0.2
Fiber One (General Mills)	½ cup	61.5	0.8/0.13	14	0	0	na	100	3	9	0.5

Food	Serving Size	Calories	Fat/Sat. Fat (gm)	Fiber (gm)	Flavonoids (mg)	Carotenoids (mcg or mg)	PE (mcg or mg)	Folate (mcg)	Selenium (mcg)	Vit. C (mg)	Vit. E (IUs)
Frosted Bran (Kellogg's)	⅔ cup	101	0.3/0.03	3.4	0	0	na	90	3	14.5	0.34
Fruit & Fibre (Post)	1 cup	212	3/0.4	5	na	0	na	100	na	0	na
Fruit Granola, lowfat (Nature's Valley)	⅔ cup	212	3/0.4	3.4	na	0	na	7	9.5	0	1.2
Fruit N' Nut Granola (Nature's Valley)	⅔ cup	253	11/2	3.4	na	0	na	10	9.5	0	9
Granola, homemade	1 cup	570	30/6	13	0	na	na	105	25	1.7	23.5
Granola, lowfat (Kellogg's)	½ cup	213	3/0.5	3.2	0	0	na	110	9.5	1.65	0
Grape-Nuts (Post)	½ cup	208	1/0.2	5	0	0	na	100	na	0	na
Grape-Nuts Flakes (Post)	¾ cup	106	0.8/0.17	2.5	0	0	na	100	na	0	na
Great Grains Raisin, Date & Pecan (Post)	⅔ cup	203	4.5/0.6	4	na	na	na	100	na	0.05	na
Heartland Natural	1 cup	500	18/4.5	7	0	0	na	64	20	1	1
Honey Bran	1 cup	119	0.7/0.25	4	0	0	na	23.5	2.5	18.5	1.2
Kasha	1 cup	154	1/0.2	4.5	0	0	na	23.5	4	0	0.6
King Vitaman (Quaker)	1¼ cup	120	1/0.25	1.2	0	0	na	104	6	12.4	3
Kix (General Mills)	1⅓ cup	114	0.6/0.17	0.8	0	0	na	336	6	15	0.12
Kretschmer Honey Crunch Wheat Germ Cereal (Quaker)	1⅓ cup	52	1/0.15	1.5	0	0	na	47	8	0	4.6
Life (Quaker)	1 cup	167	1.8/0.3	3	0	11 mcg (BC)	na	147	10.4	0	0.3
Mueslix (Kellogg's)	⅔ cup	200	3.2/0.4	3.7	0	0	na	110	9.5	0	8.3
Multi-Bran Chex	1 cup	165	1.2/0.2	6.4	0	0	na	88	4	5	0

Food	Serving Size	Calories	Fat/Sat. Fat (gm)	Fiber (gm)	Flavonoids (mg)	Carotenoids (mcg or mg)	PE (mcg or mg)	Folate (mcg)	Selenium (mcg)	Vit. C (mg)	Vit. E (IUs)
Multi-Grain Flakes (Kellogg's)	1 cup	104	0.36/0.03	3	0	0	na	90	3	0	4.5
Nutri-Grain (Kellogg's)	¾ cup	100	1/0.06	4	0	0	na	90	3	15	8
Oat Bran Cereal (Quaker)	1¼ cup	213	3/0.5	6	0	0	na	104	17	6	3
Oat Life (Quaker)	¾ cup	121	1.3/0.24	2	0	0	na	107	7.5	0	0.24
Product 19 (Kellogg's)	1 cup	110	0.4/0.03	1	0	0	na	659	3.6	60	33
Puffed Rice	1 cup	56	0.07/0.01	0.24	0	0	na	2.7	1.5	0	na
Puffed Wheat	1 cup	44	0.14/0.02	0.5	0	0	na	4	15	0	na
Quisp (Quaker)	1 cup	109	1.5/0.4	0.7	0	0	na	102	5.5	0	0.2
Raisin Bran (Kellogg's)	1 cup	186	1.5/0	8	0	0	na	122	4	0	0.8
Raisin Bran (Post)	1 cup	187	1/0.17	8	0	0	na	100	na	0	na
Raisin Nut Bran (General Mills)	1 cup	209	4.4/0.7	5	0	0	na	100	4	0	3
Rice Chex (General Mills)	1¼ cup	117	0.16/0.04	0.23	0	0	na	341	1	6	0
Rice Krispies (Kellogg's)	1¼ cup	124	0.36/0.13	0.36	0	0	na	116.5	5	16.5	0.06
Shredded Wheat (Post)	2 biscuits	156	0.5/0.09	5.3	0	0	na	20	na	0	na
Shredded Wheat, spoon-sized (Post)	1 cup	167	0.5/0.1	5.6	0	0	na	21	na	0	na
Shredded Wheat and Bran (Post)	1¼ cup	197	0.8/0.1	8	0	0	na	27	na	0	na
Smart Start (Kellogg's)	¾ cup	103	0.5/0.3	1	0	0	na	100	13	15	0.2
Special K (Kellogg's)	1 cup	115	0.3/0	1	0	0	na	93	17	15	0.12
Team (General Mills)	1 cup	113	1/0.2	1.7	0	0	na	202	5	6	0.24

Food	Serving Size	Calories	Fat/Sat. Fat (gm)	Fiber (gm)	Flavonoids (mg)	Carotenoids (mcg or mg)	PE (mcg or mg)	Folate (mcg)	Selenium (mcg)	Vit. C (mg)	Vit. E (IUs)
Toasted Oatmeal, Honey Nut (Quaker)	1 cup	191	2.7/0.5	3.3	0	0	na	100	8.5	6	3
Total (General Mills)	¾ cup	105	0.7/0.2	2.7	0	0	na	675	1.4	60	35
Total Corn Flakes (General Mills)	1⅓ cup	112	0.5/0.15	0.75	0	0	na	676	1.5	60	45
Total Raisin Bran (General Mills)	1 cup	178	1/0.23	5	0	0	na	673	4	0	45
Wheat Chex (Ralston)	1 cup	104	0.7/0.12	3.3	0	0	na	407	1.5	3.6	0.66
Wheaties (General Mills)	1 cup	110	1/0.2	2	0	0	na	100	1.4	15	0.55
CEREALS/HOT CEREALS											
Corn grits, prepared:											
Instant	1 cup	159	0.5/0.05	2.2	0	0	na	83	7.6	0	0.07
Regular, white	1 cup	145	0.5/0.07	0.5	0	0	na	75	na	0	0.18
Regular, yellow	1 cup	145	0.5/0.07	0.5	0	0	na	75	na	0	0.18
Cream of rice	1 cup	127	0.24/0.05	0.25	0	0	na	7.3	na	0	na
Cream of wheat:											
Instant	1 cup	154	0.5/0.07	3	0	0	na	150	na	0	na
Regular	1 cup	133	0.5/0.08	1.8	0	0	na	45	na	0	0.05
With fruit & maple	1 pkt.	132	0.5/0.06	0.5	na	0	na	100	na	0	na
Farina	1 cup	116.5	0.23/0.02	3.3	0	0	na	54	na	0	na
Malt-O-Meal	1 cup	171	1/0.2	2	0	0	na	19	34	0	1.4
Multi-Grain (Roman Meal)	1 cup	147	1/0.13	8	0	0	na	24	na	0	na

96

Food	Serving Size	Calories	Fat/Sat. (gm)	Fiber (gm)	Flavonoids (mg)	Carotenoids (mcg or mg)	PE (mcg or mg)	Folate (mcg)	Selenium (mcg)	Vit. C (mg)	Vit. E (IUs)
Nutrition for Women, oats & soy (Quaker)	1 pkt.	160	2/0.5	3	0	0	na	140	na	0	8
Oat bran	½ cup	146	3/0.6	6	0	0	na	15	na	0	0.23
Oatmeal:											
Flavored	1 packet	110	1.6/0.3	3.7	0	0	na	6	12	18.6	1.6
Instant	½ cup	152	2.5/0.4	4.5	0	0	na	118	14	0	0.45
Regular	½ cup	98	1.6/0.3	2.7	0	0	na	6	8.7	0	0.3
Wheatena	1 cup	136	1.2/0.2	6.6	0	0	na	17	na	0	1.3
CHEESE											
Blue or Roquefort	1 oz.	99	8/5	0	0	13 mcg (BC)	0	10	4	0	0.3
Brick	1 oz.	105	8.4/5.3	0	0	22 mcg (BC)	0	6	4	0	0.15
Brie	1 oz.	93	7.8/5	0	0	15 mcg (BC)	0	18	4	0	0.3
Camembert	1 oz.	84	7/4	0	0	20 mcg (BC)	0	17	4	0	0.3
Cheddar	1 oz.	110	9/6	0	0	30 mcg (BC)	0	5	4	0	0.15
Cheddar, lowfat	1 oz.	48	2/1.2	0	0	6.6 mcg (BC)	0	5	4	0	0.15
Colby	1 oz.	110	9/6	0	0	30 mcg (BC)	0	5	4	0	0.15
Cottage cheese:											
1% fat	½ cup	82	1/0.7	0	0	na	0	14	10	0	0.18
2% fat	½ cup	101	2/1.3	0	0	na	0	15	11.5	0	0.09
Creamed, large or small curd	½ cup	117	5/3	0	0	na	0	14	10	0	0.2
Nonfat (Light n' Lively)	½ cup	90	0/0	0	0	na	0	na	na	0	na

Food	Serving Size	Calories	Fat/Sat. Fat (gm)	Fiber (gm)	Flavonoids (mg)	Carotenoids (mcg or mg)	PE (mcg or mg)	Folate (mcg)	Selenium (mcg)	Vit. C (mg)	Vit. E (IUs)
With fruit	½ cup	140	3.8/2.4	0	0	6.6 mcg (BC)	0	11	8	0	0.15
Cream cheese:											
Lowfat	1 tbsp.	35	2.6/1.7	0	0	11 mcg (BC)	0	3	0.6	0	0.15
Nonfat	1 tbsp.	15	0.2/0.1	0	0	0	0	5.8	0.8	0	0
Regular	1 tbsp.	51	5/3	0	0	na	0	2	0.35	0	0.2
Edam or Gouda	1 oz.	100	8/5	0	0	18 mcg (BC)	0	5	4	0	0.3
Feta	1 oz.	74	6/4	0	0	5 mcg (BC)	0	9	4	0	0
Gruyere	1 oz.	115	9/5	0	0	55 mcg (BC)	0	3	4	0	0.15
Gorgonzola	1 oz.	99	8/5	0	0	13 mcg (BC)	0	10	4	0	0.3
Limburger	1 oz.	92	7.6/4.7	0	0	25 mcg (BC)	0	16	4	0	0.3
Monterey Jack	1 oz.	104.5	8.5/5.3	0	0	52 mcg (BC)	0	5	4	0	0.15
Monterey Jack, lowfat	1 oz.	88	6/4	0	0	0	0	5	4	0	0.3
Mozzarella, whole milk	1 oz.	79	6/3.7	0	0	21.6 mcg (BC)	0	2	4	0	0.15
Mozzarella, part skim	1 oz.	78	5/3	0	0	17 mcg (BC)	0	3	4.6	0	0.15
Mozzarella, fat-free	1 oz.	42	0/0	0.5	0	5 mcg (BC)	0	3	5.3	0	0
Muenster	1 oz.	103	8.4/5.4	0	0	22 mcg (BC)	0	3.4	4	0	0.15
Parmesan or Romano, dry grated	1 tbsp.	23	1.5/1	0	0	9.6 mcg (BC)	0	0.4	1.3	0	0
Parmesan or Romano, hard	1 oz.	111	7.3/4.7	0	0	44 mcg (BC)	0	2	6.4	0	0.3
Provolone	1 oz.	98	7.5/5	0	0	8.4 mcg (BC)	0	3	4	0	0.15
Ricotta:											
Light (Sargento)	½ cup	60	2.5/1.5	0	0	na		na	na	0	na
Lowfat (Frigo)	¼ cup	64	2/1	0	0	na		na	na	0	na

Food	Serving Size	Calories	Fat/Sat. Fat (gm)	Fiber (gm)	Flavonoids (mg)	Carotenoids (mcg or mg)	PE (mcg or mg)	Folate (mcg)	Selenium (mcg)	Vit. C (mg)	Vit. E (IUs)
Nonfat (Frigo)	¼ cup	47.5	0.4/0.2	0	0	na	0	na	na	0	na
Part-skim	¼ cup	80	5/3	0	0	na	0	na	na	0	na
Whole milk	¼ cup	108	8/5	0	0	na	0	7.5	9	0	0.3
Swiss	1 oz.	105	7.7/5	0	0	13 mcg (BC)	0	1.8	3.6	0	0.15
Swiss, lowfat	1 oz.	50	1.4/0.9	0	0	13 mcg (BC)	0	1.7	3.6	0	0.15
CHEESE PRODUCTS											
American cheese, singles	1 oz.	90	7/4	0	0	53 mcg (BC)	0	na	na	na	na
American cheese food, spread, from jar	1 oz.	83	6/4	0	0	39 mcg (BC)	0	2	3	0	0.3
American cheese, nonfat	1 slice	25	0/0	0	0	na	0	na	na	6	na
Cheese food (Velveeta)	1 oz.	80	6/4	0	0	na	0	na	na	na	na
Cheese food, reduced fat (Velveeta)	1 oz.	62	3/2	0	0	na	0	na	na	na	na
Cheese food, Swiss (Velveeta)	1 oz.	100	7/4	0	0	na	0	na	na	na	na
CHICKEN											
Fried, batter dipped:											
Breast	1 breast	218	11/3	0.25	0	0	0	12.6	23.5	0	1.4
Drumstick	1 drumstick	115	6.7/1.8	0.13	0	0	0	7.7	9.4	0	0
Thigh	1 thigh	238	14/4	0.26	0	0	0	16	20	0	0
Wing	1 wing	94	6/1.7	0.09	0	0	0	5	7.5	0	0

99

Food	Serving Size	Calories	Fat/Sat. Fat (gm)	Fiber (gm)	Flavonoids (mg)	Carotenoids (mcg or mg)	PE (mcg or mg)	Folate (mcg)	Selenium (mcg)	Vit. C (mg)	Vit. E (IUs)
Fried, flour coated:											
Breast	1 breast	131	5/1.5	0.06	0	0	0	3.5	14	0	0
Drumstick	1 drumstick	71	4/1	0.03	0	0	0	3	5.3	0	0
Thigh	1 thigh	162	9/2.5	0.06	0	0	0	7.4	12.3	0	0
Wing	1 wing	61	4/1.15	0.02	0	0	0	1.14	4	0	0
Ground:											
Patty, cooked	1 patty (4 oz.)	143	8/2.3	0	0	0	0	3	14	0	0.3
Roasted:											
Breast (meat only)	1 breast	86	2/0.5	0	0	0	0	2	14	0	0.2
Breast (meat & skin)	1 breast	114	4.5/1.2	0	0	0	0	2.3	14	0	0.2
Dark meat	1 cup	269	12.6/3.4	0	0	0	0	9	24	0	0.5
Leg	1 leg	109	5/1.3	0	0	0	0	4.5	12.6	0	18
Light meat	1 cup	242	6/1.7	0	0	0	0	5.6	35	0	0.5
Thigh	1 thigh	91	6/1.6	0	0	0	0	2.6	7	0	0.15
Wing	1 wing	61	4/1.14	0	0	0	0	0.6	4.6	0	0.08
Canned, boneless	1 can (5 oz.)	230	10/2.8	0	0	0	0	2.5	23	0	0.6
Giblets:											
Fried	1 cup	402	19.5/5.5	0	0	0	0	550	151	13	0
Simmered	1 cup	228	7/2	0	0	0	0	545	136	12	3
Liver:											
Simmered	1 cup	220	7.6/2.6	0	0	0	0	1,078	140	22	3

Food	Serving Size	Calories	Fat/Sat. Fat (gm)	Fiber (gm)	Flavonoids (mg)	Carotenoids (mcg or mg)	PE (mcg or mg)	Folate (mcg)	Selenium (mcg)	Vit. C (mg)	Vit. E (IUs)
CONDIMENTS											
A-1 Steak Sauce	1 tbsp.	18	0/0	0	na	89 mcg (BC)	na	na	na	na	na
Au jus gravy, canned	¼ cup	9.5	0.12/0.06	0	na	0	na	1.2	0.24	0.6	na
Au jus gravy mix, prep. as directed	¼ cup	10	0/0	0	na	0	na	na	na	na	na
Barbecue sauce	1 tbsp.	15	0.1/0	0.1	na	83 mcg (BC)	na	na	na	na	na
Bernaise sauce	1 tbsp.	96	10/0	0	na	na	na	na	na	na	na
Beef gravy, canned	¼ cup	31	1.4/0.7	0.23	na	0	na	1	0.6	0	0.05
Beef gravy, nonfat	¼ cup	15	0/0	0	na	0	na	na	na	na	na
Brown gravy, canned or jar	¼ cup	25	1/0	0	na	0	na	na	na	na	na
Brown gravy mix, prep. w/ water	¼ cup	16	0/0	0	na	0	na	na	na	na	na
Catsup	1 tbsp.	15	0/0	0	na	91 mcg (BC) 2.6 mg (LYC)	na	na	na	1.2	na
Catsup, light (Heinz)	1 tbsp.	8	0/0	0.2	na	na	na	na	na	na	na
Cheese sauce, ready to serve (Nestlé)	¼ cup	133	11/5	0.6	0	0	0	3	na	0.06	0.4
Chicken gravy, canned	¼ cup	47	3.4/0.8	0.24	na	0	na	1.2	0.5	0	0.14
Chicken gravy, mix, prep. w/ water	¼ cup	25	1/0	0	na	0	na	na	na	na	na
Chili sauce (Del Monte)	1 tbsp.	20	0/0	0	na	70 mcg (BC)	na	na	na	1.2	na
Cocktail sauce (Golden Dipt)	1 tbsp.	20	0/0	0	na	77 mcg (BC)	na	na	na	na	na

101

Food	Serving Size	Calories	Fat/Sat. Fat (gm)	Fiber (gm)	Flavonoids (mg)	Carotenoids (mcg or mg)	PE (mcg or mg)	Folate (mcg)	Selenium (mcg)	Vit. C (mg)	Vit. E (IUs)
Enchilada sauce	¼ cup	20	1/0	0.4	na	130 mcg (BC)	na	na	na	2.7	na
Hollandaise sauce	1 tbsp.	96	10/0	0	na	37 mcg (BC)	na	na	na	na	na
Horseradish	1 tbsp.	10	0/0	0	na	0	na	na	na	na	na
Horseradish sauce	1 tbsp.	74	7/0	0	na	17 mcg (BC)	na	na	na	na	na
Mushroom gravy, canned	¼ cup	25	1/0	0	na	0	na	na	na	na	na
Mushroom gravy, creamy	¼ cup	20	1/0	0	na	0	na	na	na	0	na
Mushroom gravy, mix, prep. w/ water	¼ cup	20	1/0	0	na	0	na	na	na	na	na
Mustard, brown	1 tbsp.	14	1/0	0	na	0	na	na	na	na	na
Mustard (Grey Poupon)	1 tbsp.	19	1/0.06	0.3	na	0	na	0.3	na	0.12	na
Mustard, yellow	1 tbsp.	10	0.5/0	0.5	na	0	na	1	2	0.5	0.13
Onion gravy, mix, prep. w/ water	¼ cup	25	1/0	0	na	na	na	na	na	na	na
Pesto sauce (Contadina)	¼ cup	310	30/5	0	na	288 mcg (BC)	na	na	na	0	na
Pesto sauce w/ sun-dried tomato (Contadina)	¼ cup	250	24/4	3	na	na	na	na	na	na	na
Picante sauce, mild (Old El Paso)	2 tbsp.	10	0/0	0	na	127 mcg (BC)	na	na	na	0	na
Pork gravy mix, prep. w/ water	¼ cup	20	1/0	0	na	na	na	na	na	na	na
Salsa, mild	2 tbsp.	7	0.1/0	0.5	na	127 mcg (BC)	na	na	na	3	na
Salsa, black bean	2 tbsp.	10	0/0	1	na	na	na	na	na	na	na

102

Food	Serving Size	Calories	Fat/Sat. Fat (gm)	Fiber (gm)	Flavonoids (mg)	Carotenoids (mcg or mg)	PE (mcg or mg)	Folate (mcg)	Selenium (mcg)	Vit. C (mg)	Vit. E (IUs)
Salsa, chunky, mild or medium (Old El Paso)	2 tbsp.	15	0/0	1	na	127 mcg (BC)	na	na	na	0	na
Salsa, green chili, mild	2 tbsp.	8	0.08/0	0.12	na	27 mcg (BC)	na	na	na	4	na
Salsa, green jalapeño	2 tbsp.	8	2/0	0	na	na	na	na	na	na	na
Stroganoff sauce	¼ cup	30	2/0	0	na	na	na	na	na	na	na
Sweet and sour sauce (Kikkoman)	1 tbsp.	17.5	0/0	0	na	0	na	na	na	0	na
Sweet and sour sauce (La Choy)	1 tbsp.	29	0.1/0	0	na	0	na	na	na	0	na
Tabasco sauce	¼ tsp.	0.15	t/t	t	na	t	na	t	na	0.05	na
Taco sauce, canned (Old El Paso)	2 tbsp.	15	0/0	1	na	127 mcg (BC)	na	na	na	na	na
Tartar sauce (Hellman's)	1 tbsp.	70	8/1	0	na	8 mcg (BC)	na	na	na	na	na
Tartar sauce, egg-free	1 tbsp.	38	4/0	0	na	na	na	na	na	na	na
Tartar sauce, nonfat	1 tbsp.	10	0/0	0	na	8 mcg (BC)	na	na	na	na	na
Teriyaki sauce (La Choy)	1 tbsp.	16.5	t/0	0.5	na	0	na	na	na	0	na
Turkey gravy, canned	¼ cup	30	1.25/0.37	0.24	na	0	na	1.2	0.36	0	0.05
Turkey gravy, nonfat (Heinz)	¼ cup	15	0/0	0	na	0	na	na	na	na	na
Turkey gravy mix, prep. w/ water	¼ cup	22	1/0	0	na	0	na	na	na	na	na
White sauce, homemade	½ cup	92	7/1.7	0.1	na	62 mcg (BC)	na	5	2.5	0.5	1.3
Worcestershire sauce	1 tbsp.	6	0/0	0	na	11 mcg (BC)	na	na	na	na	na

CRACKERS

Food	Serving Size	Calories	Fat/Sat. Fat (gm)	Fiber (gm)	Flavonoids (mg)	Carotenoids (mcg or mg)	PE (mcg or mg)	Folate (mcg)	Selenium (mcg)	Vit. C (mg)	Vit. E (IUs)
Amaranth crackers, nonfat	8 crackers	100	0/0	3	na	na	na	5	na	0	na
Bran crackers (Nabisco Bran Thins)	7 crackers	60	3/1	0	na	na	na	na	na	na	na
Brown rice crackers (Eden)	5 crackers	120	2/0	2	na	0	na	na	na	0	na
Butter crackers (Town House)	4 crackers	70	4/1	0	na	na	na	na	na	na	na
Cheese-flavored crackers, nonfat (Health Valley)	5 crackers	50	0/0	2	na	t (BC)	na	na	na	2	na
Cheez-Its, reduced fat (Sunshine)	14 crackers	59	1/0.2	0.4	na	11.4 mcg (BC)	na	16	5	0.3	0.3
Cracked pepper crackers, fat-free	4 crackers	35	0/0	0	na	0	na	9.6	0.4	0	0
Crackerbread (Crisp & Light)	1 slice	17	1/0	0	na	0	na	na	na	na	na
Crispbread (Wasa)	1 cracker	25	0/0	0	na	0	na	na	na	na	na
Crispbread, high-fiber (Ryvita)	1 cracker	23	1/0	2	na	0	na	na	na	na	na
Crispbread, multigrain (Wasa)	1 slice	45	0/0	2	na	0	na	na	na	na	na
Crispbread, Norwegian rye	1 cracker	21	0.07/t	1	na	0	na	3	2	0	0.12
Graham cracker	4 pieces	118	3/0.4	1	na	0	na	13	na	0	na
Graham snacks, cinnamon, fat-free (Snackwell)	7 crackers	53	0.1/0	0.6	na	0	na	10	3.4	0	0

Food	Serving Size	Calories	Fat/Sat. Fat (gm)	Fiber (gm)	Flavonoids (mg)	Carotenoids (mcg or mg)	PE (mcg or mg)	Folate (mcg)	Selenium (mcg)	Vit. C (mg)	Vit. E (IUs)
Herb cracker, nonfat (Health Valley)	1 serving	40	0/0	2	na	na	na	na	na	na	na
Matzoh	1 matzoh	115	2/0.4	0.3	na	0	na	10	na	0	na
Matzoh, dietetic	1 matzoh	91	0.4/0	0.1	na	0	na	10	na	0	na
Matzoh, whole wheat	1 matzoh	100	0.4/0.07	3.4	na	0	na	10	21	na	0.6
Melba toast, bran	1 cracker	16	0.4/0.1	0.2	na	0	na	6	na	0	na
Melba toast, plain	1 cracker	19.5	0.16/0.02	0.3	na	0	na	15	2	0	t
Melba toast rounds	4 rounds	47	0.4/0	0.8	na	0	na	6.6	4	0	0
Melba toast, wheat	1 cracker	19	0.12/0.08	0.4	na	0	na		3	0	na
Melba toast, whole grain	1 cracker	16	0.4/0.1	0.2	na	0	na	na	na	0	na
Multigrain cracker, stoned wheat (Health Valley)	13 crackers	120	5/0	3	na	0	na	na	na	na	na
Oat cracker (Oat Thins)	18 crackers	140	6/1	2	na	0	na	na	na	0.6	na
Oyster crackers	17 crackers	60	1.5/0	0.5	na	0	na	na	na	0.6	na
Rice cracker (Weight Watchers)	2 crackers	30	0/0	0	na	0	na	na	na	0	na
Ritz cracker (Nabisco)	1 serving	79	4/0.6	0.3	na	0	na	10	na	0	na
Ry-Crisp	2 crackers	60	0/0	4	na	0	na	na	na	0	na
Saltines (Zesta)	5 crackers	60	2/1	0	na	0	na	18.5	2	0	0
Saltines, multigrain (Premium)	5 crackers	60	1.5/0	1	na	0	na	na	na	na	na
Saltines, nonfat	6 crackers	118	0.5/0.07	1	na	0	na	23	4	0	0.03
Saltines, wheat (Zesta)	5 crackers	60	2/1	0	na	0	na	10	7	0	t

Food	Serving Size	Calories	Fat/Sat. Fat (gm)	Fiber (gm)	Flavonoids (mg)	Carotenoids (mcg or mg)	PE (mcg or mg)	Folate (mcg)	Selenium (mcg)	Vit. C (mg)	Vit. E (IUs)
Sesame cracker (Keebler)	4 crackers	60	3/1	0	na	0	na	na	na	na	na
Sesame sticks	¼ cup	133	9/0	0.1	na	t (BC)	na	na	na	na	na
Soda cracker	4 crackers	70	1/0	0	na	0	na	na	na	na	na
Triscuit	4 crackers	71	3/0.5	2	na	0	na	4.5	2.4	0	1
Triscuit, whole wheat & bran	4 crackers	70	3/0.4	1.6	na	0	na	5	2.4	0	1.2
Triscuit, whole wheat, reduced fat	4 crackers	65	1.7/0.3	2	na	0	na	5	11	0	0.6
Vegetable cracker	3 crackers	70	3/1.5	0	na	na	na	na	na	na	na
Waverly Wafers	4 crackers	80	4/0.8	0.4	na	0	na	12	1	0	1
Wafer cracker (Carr's)	2 crackers	25	1/0	0	na	0	na	na	na	na	na
Wheat cracker (Wheatsworth)	4 crackers	57	2.5/0.6	0.5	na	0	na	5.3	0.76	0	0.6
Wheat Thins	8 crackers	70	3/1	0	na	0	na	10	1.6	0	na
Wheat Thins, reduced fat	8 crackers	58	1.6/0	0.8	na	0	na	8	5	0	0
DIET AND SPORTS PRODUCTS/BARS											
Apple breakfast bar (Ultra Slim•Fast)	1 bar	160	0/0	1	na	1.7 mg (BC)	na	100	na	6	na
Apple cinnamon bar (PowerBar)	1 bar	230	2.5/0.5	3	na	na	na	400	na	60	30
Banana energy bar (PowerBar)	1 bar	230	2/1	3	na	na	na	400	na	60	67.5

Food	Serving Size	Calories	Fat/Sat. Fat (gm)	Fiber (gm)	Flavonoids (mg)	Carotenoids (mcg or mg)	PE (mcg or mg)	Folate (mcg)	Selenium (mcg)	Vit C (mg)	Vit E (IUs)
Breakfast bar (Fi-Bar)	1 bar	150	4/0	5	na	0.6 mcg (BC)	na	na	na	na	na
Breakfast bar, blueberry (Ultra Slim•Fast)	1 bar	170	0/0	2	na	na	na	100	na	6	na
Brownie bar (Ultra Slim•Fast)	1 bar	120	4/1	1	na	1.7 mg (BC)	na	40	na	6	na
Chocolate chip crunch bar (Slim•Fast)	1 bar	120	4/2	2	na	1.7 mg (BC)	na	60	na	9	na
Chocolate energy bar (PowerBar)	1 bar	240	4/1	4	na	na	na	200	na	60	67.5
Diet bar, chocolate brownie (Atkins)	1 bar	230	10/3	2	na	na	na	240	na	36	18
Diet bar, chocolate coconut (Atkins)	1 bar	250	13/8	1	na	na	na	240	na	36	18
Dutch chocolate bar (Slim•Fast)	1 bar	140	5/2	2	na	1.7 mg (BC)	na	40	na	15	na
Energy bar for women, apple crunch (Viactiv)	1 bar	180	5/4	na	na	na	na	400	na	na	na
Energy bar, apple caramel (MET-Rx)	1 bar	190	3/3	1	na	na	na	200	na	78	228
Energy bar, apple cherry (CliffBar)	1 bar	250	2/1	5	na	na	na	na	na	60	67.5
Energy bar, chocolate, 40/30/30 (Complete)	1 bar	190	6/3	0	na	na	na	na	na	15	na

Food	Serving Size	Calories	Fat/Sat. Fat (gm)	Fiber (gm)	Flavonoids (mg)	Carotenoids (mcg or mg)	PE (mcg or mg)	Folate (mcg)	Selenium (mcg)	Vit. C (mg)	Vit. E (IUs)
Energy bar, chocolate chip (ClifBar)	1 bar	250	3/1	3	na	na	na	na	na	60	67.5
Meal replacement bar, coconut cream (Lean Body)	1 bar	300	7/6	0	na	na	na	320	na	54	24
Meal replacement bar, chocolate (Jenny Craig)	1 bar	220	5/4	1	na	na	na	100	na	60	30
Nutrition bar, 40/30/30 (PR*Bar)	1 bar	190	7/3	2	na	na	na	400	na	120	133.5
Nutrition bar, chocolate (Myoplex)	1 bar	340	7/2	2	na	na	na	200	na	30	33
Nutrition bar, extreme chocolate (MET-Rx)	1 bar	240	8/1	3	na	na	na	400	na	60	100.5
Peanut butter bar (Slim•Fast)	1 bar	150	5/3	2	na	1.7 mg (BC)	na	40	na	15	na
Peanut butter crunch bar (Ultra Slim•Fast)	1 bar	120	4/2	2	na	1.7 mg (BC)	na	60	na	9	na
Protein bar, chocolate (Bally)	1 bar	320	7/1.5	1	na	na	na	na	na	na	na
Protein bar, chocolate (Biox)	1 bar	290	5/4	2	na	na	na	140	30	21	24
Protein bar, chocolate chip (Pure Protein)	1 bar	290	5/4	na	na	na	na	360	na	60	27
Protein bar, double fudge chocolate (SportPharma)	1 bar	270	5/4	2	na	na	na	100	na	15	16.5
Protein bar, oatmeal (Sci Fit)	1 bar	330	6/4	1	na	na	na	360	na	54	27

108

Food	Serving Size	Calories	Fat/Sat. Fat (gm)	Fiber (gm)	Flavonoids (mg)	Carotenoids (mcg or mg)	PE (mcg or mg)	Folate (mcg)	Selenium (mcg)	Vit. C (mg)	Vit. E (IUs)
Protein bar, peanut butter (Bally)	1 bar	340	8/2	1	na	na	na	na	na	na	na
Protein bar, protein-plus (MET-Rx)	1 bar	290	8/3	1	na	na	na	400	na	120	133.5
Snack bar (Boost)	1 bar	190	7/3.5	t	na	0	na	60	0	9	4.5
Snack bar, carbo-crunch (Shaklee)	1 bar	180	4/1	0	na	na	na	120	na	18	9
Snack bar, chocolate (Ultra Slim•Fast)	1 bar	120	4/0	3	na	1.7 mg (BC)	na	na	na	na	na
Snack bar, protein (Weider)	1 bar	160	4/0	0	na	na	na	na	na	na	na
Sports bar, apple (Twinlab)	1 bar	340	5/4	0	na	na	na	100	na	15	7.5
Sports bar, chocolate (Twinlab)	1 bar	320	5/4	2	na	na	na	100	na	15	7.5
Sports bar, peanut butter (Twinlab)	1 bar	340	5/1	0	na	na	na	100	na	15	7.5
DIET AND SPORTS PRODUCTS/BEVERAGES											
Chocolate or vanilla drink, canned (Ensure)	8 fl. oz.	250	6/0.5	0	0	0	na	100	14	30	3.75
Chocolate or vanilla drink, canned (Ensure Plus)	8 fl. oz.	360	11/1	0	0	529 mcg (BC)	na	100	14	30	3.75
Chocolate or vanilla drink w/ fiber, canned (Ensure Fiber)	8 fl. oz.	250	6/0.5	3	0	0	na	100	14	30	3.75

109

Food	Serving Size	Calories	Fat/Sat. Fat (gm)	Fiber (gm)	Flavonoids (mg)	Carotenoids (mcg or mg)	PE (mcg or mg)	Folate (mcg)	Selenium (mcg)	Vit. C (mg)	Vit. E (IUs)
Chocolate or vanilla drink, canned (Sustacal)	8 fl. oz.	240	5.5/0	0	0	0	na	na	na	na	na
Chocolate fudge shake, prep.w/ skim milk (Ultra Slim•Fast)	8 fl. oz.	200	2.6/1	5	0	0	na	120	na	30	na
Chocolate shake (Slim•Fast)	8 fl. oz.	190	1/0.8	2	0	0	na	120	na	21	na
Chocolate Super Mega Mass Weight Gainer 2000 (Weider)	8 fl. oz.	334	3/0	0	0	0	na	47	0	12	34.5
Dynamic Muscle Builder, prep. w/ skim milk (Weider)	8 fl. oz.	206	0.3/0.6	0.75	0	0	na	150	na	22.5	11
Fat Burner System Drink, prep. w/ skim milk (Weider)	8 fl. oz.	146	1/0	2	0	0	na	na	na	22.5	na
Fiber Drink Mix (Shaklee)	1 tbsp.	20	1/0	3	na	na	na	na	na	na	na
Gelatin Drink Mix, orange flavor, prep. w/ water (Genesis Nutrition)	1 pkt.	67	0.3/0.02	0	na	na	na	0	0.4	50.5	na
Milk & egg protein supplement (Genesis Nutrition)	1 tbsp.	39	0/0	na	na	na	na	na	na	na	na
Nutra Start Vanilla Shake (Slim•Fast)	1 shake	210	2.5/0	5	0	0	na	100	na	60	na
Nutrition drink (Boost)	8 fl. oz.	240	4/0.5	0	0	0.3 mg (BC)	na	140	14	60	30

Food	Serving Size	Calories	Fat/Sat. Fat (gm)	Fiber (gm)	Flavonoids (mg)	Carotenoids (mcg or mg)	PE (mcg or mg)	Folate (mcg)	Selenium (mcg)	Vit. C (mg)	Vit. E (IUs)
Nutrition drink w/ protein, strawberry, vanilla flavors (MET-Rx)	3 scoops	210	1/1	0	0	na	na	na	na	0	na
Nutrition drink, muscle builder (EAS)	3 tbsp.	100	1/1	1	0	na	na	na	na	na	na
Nutrition drink, vanilla (Lean Body)	1 pkt.	300	2/1	1	0	na	na	200	na	30	15
Nutrition shake, chocolate (SportPharma)	3 scoops	450	1/1	1	0	na	na	200	na	30	15
Nutrition shake, whey, all flavors (Twinlab)	1 pkt.	300	2/1	0	0	na	na	200	na	30	30
Performance Shaper Diet, prep. w/ skim milk (Weider)	8 fl. oz.	180	0.7/0	0.75	0	na	na	150	na	22.5	10
Pure egg protein, prep. w/ skim milk (Weider)	8 fl. oz.	150	0/0	0	0	0	0	na	na	0	na
Slim Plan Vanilla Drink Mix (Shaklee)	½ cup	210	3/0	4	0	na	na	140	na	21	na
Sports drink mix, banana (Nature's Way)	1 scoop	94	0/0	2	0	na	na	na	na	na	na
Sports shake meal replacement, all flavors (Nutrament)	12 fl. oz.	360	10/0	0	0	0	na	na	na	na	na

Food	Serving Size	Calories	Fat/Sat. Fat (gm)	Fiber (gm)	Flavonoids (mg)	Carotenoids (mcg or mg)	PE (mcg or mg)	Folate (mcg)	Selenium (mcg)	Vit. C (mg)	Vit. E (IUs)
DINNERS/AMY'S KITCHEN (VEGETARIAN MEALS)											
Black bean enchilada	1 meal	250	8/1	5	na	na	na	na	na	na	na
Cannelloni	1 meal	330	12/8	6	na	na	na	na	na	na	na
Cheese enchilada	1 meal	330	14/7	6	na	na	na	na	na	na	na
Chili and cornbread	1 meal	320	6/2	8	na	na	na	na	na	na	na
Country dinner	1 meal	380	12/4	9	na	na	na	na	na	na	na
Veggie loaf	1 meal	260	5/0.5	7	na	na	na	na	na	na	na
DINNERS/HEALTHY CHOICE											
Beef pot roast	1 meal	330	9/3	8	na	na	na	na	na	**18**	na
Beef stroganoff	1 meal	330	9/3	7	na	na	na	na	na	12	na
Beef tips portobello	1 meal	310	9/3	7	na	na	na	na	na	12	na
Blackened chicken	1 meal	320	6/2	5	na	na	na	na	na	**48**	na
Charbroiled beef patty	1 meal	310	9/3	4	na	na	na	na	na	0	na
Chicken broccoli Alfredo	1 meal	300	7/3	2	na	na	na	na	na	12	na
Chicken enchiladas	1 meal	270	6/3	6	na	na	na	na	na	**18**	na
Chicken parmigiana	1 meal	310	8/2	6	na	na	na	na	na	0	na
Chicken teriyaki	1 meal	270	6/2	3	na	na	na	na	na	0	na
Country breaded chicken	1 meal	380	8/2	7	na	na	na	na	na	0	na
Country herb chicken	1 meal	280	6/3	6	na	na	na	na	na	**18**	na
Grilled turkey breast	1 meal	260	5/2	5	na	na	na	na	na	**21**	na
Herb baked fish	1 meal	360	8/2	5	na	na	na	na	na	0	na
Honey glazed chicken	1 meal	320	6/2	4	na	na	na	na	na	3.6	na

Food	Serving Size	Calories	Fat/Sat. Fat (gm)	Fiber (gm)	Flavonoids (mg)	Carotenoids (mcg or mg)	PE (mcg or mg)	Folate (mcg)	Selenium (mcg)	Vit. C (mg)	Vit. E (IUs)
Lemon pepper fish	1 meal	320	7/2	5	na	na	na	na	na	30	na
Meatloaf	1 meal	330	7/3.5	6	na	na	na	na	na	42	na
Mesquite beef w/ barbecue sauce	1 meal	320	9/3	5	na	na	na	na	na	9	na
Mesquite chicken BBQ	1 meal	290	5/2	4	na	na	na	na	na	6	na
Oven roasted beef	1 meal	280	7/2.5	6	na	na	na	na	na	6	na
Roasted chicken breast	1 meal	230	6/3	4	na	na	na	na	na	3.6	na
Salisbury steak	1 meal	330	7/3	6	na	na	na	na	na	12	na
Sesame chicken	1 meal	330	8/2	5	na	na	na	na	na	15	na
Stuffed pasta shells	1 meal	370	6/3	5	na	na	na	na	na	5	na
Sweet and sour chicken	1 meal	360	7/2	3	na	na	na	na	na	30	na
Traditional turkey breasts	1 meal	320	5/2	5	na	na	na	na	na	6	na
DINNERS/LEAN CUISINE (HEARTY PORTIONS MEALS)											
Beef stroganoff	1 meal	350	9/3	9	na	na	na	na	na	6	na
Cheese and spinach manicotti	1 meal	350	8/3	6	na	na	na	na	na	9	na
Chicken and barbecue	1 meal	370	6/1	6	na	na	na	na	na	12	na
Chicken fettuccini	1 meal	400	9/4.5	4	na	na	na	na	na	36	na
Chicken florentine	1 meal	380	7/3	6	na	na	na	na	na	15	na
Glazed chicken	1 meal	360	8/1.5	2	na	na	na	na	na	3.6	na
Grilled chicken and penne pasta	1 meal	360	7/3	5	na	na	na	na	na	9	na

113

Food	Serving Size	Calories	Fat/Sat. Fat (gm)	Fiber (gm)	Flavonoids (mg)	Carotenoids (mcg or mg)	PE (mcg or mg)	Folate (mcg)	Selenium (mcg)	Vit. C (mg)	Vit. E (IUs)
Jumbo rigatoni w/ meatballs	1 meal	440	9/3.5	7	na	na	na	na	na	24	na
Oriental glazed chicken	1 meal	370	2/0.5	4	na	na	na	na	na	27	na
Roasted chicken	1 meal	330	5/1	4	na	na	na	na	na	48	na
Roasted turkey breast	1 meal	320	6/1	6	na	na	na	na	na	3.6	na
Salisbury steak	1 meal	300	6/3	8	na	na	na	na	na	6	na
DINNERS/MRS. PAUL'S											
Shrimp primavera w/ pasta	1 meal	282	5.2/1.6	4.5	na	5 mg (BC)	na	93	40	24	2
DINNERS/WEIGHT WATCHERS											
Barbecue chicken	1 meal	217	4.4/1	na	na	na	na	na	na	21.5	na
Chicken cordon bleu	1 meal	223	9/5	3	na	3.8 mg (BC)	na	37	17	14	1.8
Turkey medallions	1 meal	214	1.7/0.4	3	na	na	na	na	na	na	na
Veal parmigiana	1 meal	190	8.6/4.6	2	na	513 mcg (BC)	na	27	9	14	2
DIPS											
Avocado	2 tbsp.	46	4.4/0.7	1.4	na	104 mcg (BC)	na	18	0.1	2.4	0.6
Baba ghanoush (Eggplant dip)	2 tbsp.	47	4/0.5	0.8	na	21 mcg (BC)	na	9	0.24	2.5	0.34
Bacon and horseradish	2 tbsp.	70	6/3	0	na	na	na	na	2	na	na
Bean	2 tbsp.	40	1/0.5	2.4	na	60 mcg (BC)	na	24	2	0–5	0.6
Black bean	2 tbsp.	20	0/0	1	na	na	na	na	na	0	na
Black bean, nonfat (Tostitos)	2 tbsp.	30	0/0	2	na	na	na	na	na	na	na
Bleu cheese	2 tbsp.	50	4/2	0	0	na	na	na	na	na	na

114

Food	Serving Size	Calories	Fat/Sat. Fat (gm)	Fiber (gm)	Flavonoids (mg)	Carotenoids (mcg or mg)	PE (mcg or mg)	Folate (mcg)	Selenium (mcg)	Vit. C (mg)	Vit. E (IUs)
Cheddar cheese, nonfat	2 tbsp.	20	0/0	0	0	na	na	na	na	na	na
Clam (Kraft)	2 tbsp.	60	4/3	0	0	0	na	na	na	0	na
Creamy dill (Vegi-Dip)	2 tbsp.	60	4/0	0	na	na	na	na	na	na	na
Cucumber	2 tbsp.	50	4/3	0	na	na	na	na	na	na	na
Guacamole (Lucerne)	2 tbsp.	80	8/1.5	0	na	na	na	na	na	na	na
Hummus	2 tbsp.	51	2.6/0.4	1.6	na	3.6 mcg (BC)	na	18	0.8	na	0.6
Nacho cheese (Kraft)	2 tbsp.	55	4/2	0	na	na	na	na	na	2.4	0.6
Onion	2 tbsp.	68	6/4	0.3	na	36 mcg (BC)	na	3.5	1	0.3	0.3
Pinto bean, nonfat (Guiltless Gourmet)	2 tbsp.	27	0/0	2	na	na	na	na	na	na	na
Shrimp	2 tbsp.	74	6/4	0.1	0	21 mcg (BC)	na	3.4	3.6	0.5	0.45
Sour cream and chives	2 tbsp.	126	14/0	0	na	na	na	na	na	na	na
Spinach	2 tbsp.	54	4.4/1.4	0.4	na	447 mcg (BC)	na	13	0.6	2.5	0.75
Vegetable (Marzetti)	2 tbsp.	176	20/0	0	na	na	na	na	na	na	na
EGGS											
Egg (chicken), large	1 egg	74.5	4.5/1.5	0	0	0	0	24	15	0	0.75
White	1 large	17	0/0	0	0	0	0	1	6	0	0
Yolk	1 large	59	5/1.6	0	0	0	0	24	7.5	0	0.75
Egg, cooked:											
Fried in margarine	1 large	91.5	7/2	0	0	0	0	17.5	12	0	1
Hard-boiled, shell removed	1 large	77	5/1.6	0	0	0	0	22	15	0	0.75

Food	Serving Size	Calories	Fat/Sat. Fat (gm)	Fiber (gm)	Flavonoids (mg)	Carotenoids (mcg or mg)	PE (mcg or mg)	Folate (mcg)	Selenium (mcg)	Vit. C (mg)	Vit. E (IUs)
Poached	1 large	74.5	5/1.5	0	0	0	0	17.5	15	0	0.75
Scrambled with milk and margarine	1 large	101	7.5/2	0	0	0	0	18	14	0.12	1
Egg substitutes:											
Cholesterol-free (Healthy Choice)	⅓ cup	30	1/0	0	0	0	0	na	na	na	na
Cheese omelet Egg Beaters (Fleischmann's)	½ cup	110	5/2	0	0	0	0	na	na	na	na
Egg Beaters (Fleischmann's)	¼ cup	30	0/0	0	0	0	0	32	na	0	na
Egg Watchers (Tofutti)	¼ cup	30	0/0	0	0	0	0	40	na	na	na
Frozen Liquid Eggs (Sunny Fresh)	½ cup	130	9/3	0	0	0	0	na	na	na	na
Powdered Tofu Scrambler (Fantastic Foods)	2½ cups	60	0.5/0	3	0	0	0	1.2	na	na	na
Vegetable omelet Egg Beaters (Fleischmann's)	½ cup	50	0/0	0	0	0	0	na	na	na	na
ENTRÉES/HEALTHY CHOICE											
Beef w/ barbecue sauce and rice and beans	1 entrée	250	4/0.5	2	na	na	na	na	na	na	na
Beef macaroni	1 entrée	220	4/2	5	na	na	na	na	na	**54**	na

116

Food	Serving Size	Calories	Fat/Sat. Fat (gm)	Fiber (gm)	Flavonoids (mg)	Carotenoids (mcg or mg)	PE (mcg or mg)	Folate (mcg)	Selenium (mcg)	Vit. C (mg)	Vit. E (IUs)
Beef teriyaki	1 entrée	330	7/2.5	7	na	na	na	na	na	6	na
Beef tips, sirloin w/ mushroom sauce	1 entrée	270	6/2	4	na	na	na	na	na	0	na
Beef tips w/ spiral pasta	1 entrée	300	7/2.5	4	na	na	na	na	na	0	na
Chicken, baked w/ mashed potatoes	1 entrée	210	4.5/1.5	3	na	na	na	na	na	5	na
Chicken breast, breaded w/ macaroni and cheese	1 entrée	270	6/2.5	1	na	na	na	na	na	1.2	na
Chicken breast, grilled w/ pasta	1 entrée	240	6/2.5	4	na	na	na	na	na	6	na
Chicken breast w/ vegetables	1 entrée	230	5/2	6	na	na	na	na	na	6	na
Chicken carbonara	1 entrée	310	5/2.5	2	na	na	na	na	na	6	na
Chicken, country glazed	1 entrée	250	5/2	3	na	na	na	na	na	0	na
Chicken enchilada	1 entrée	310	7/2.5	6	na	na	na	na	na	0	na
Chicken, grilled w/ mashed potatoes	1 entrée	200	4/2	6	na	na	na	na	na	3.6	na
Chicken, grilled Sonoma	1 entrée	230	4/1	3	na	na	na	na	na	12	na
Chicken, Mandarin	1 entrée	280	3.5/0.5	4	na	na	na	na	na	9	na
Chicken olé	1 entrée	270	4/1	5	na	na	na	na	na	0	na
Chicken, oriental style	1 entrée	240	5/1.5	7	na	na	na	na	na	5	na
Chicken and pasta, homestyle	1 entrée	270	6/2.5	5	na	na	na	na	na	3.6	na

Food	Serving Size	Calories	Fat/Sat. Fat (gm)	Fiber (gm)	Flavonoids (mg)	Carotenoids (mcg or mg)	PE (mcg or mg)	Folate (mcg)	Selenium (mcg)	Vit. C (mg)	Vit. E (IUs)
Chicken piccata	1 entrée	270	5/2.5	2	na	na	na	na	na	12	na
Chicken and rice, cheesy	1 entrée	230	4/2.5	5	na	na	na	na	na	18	na
Chicken, sesame	1 entrée	240	6/2	4	na	na	na	na	na	21	na
Fettucini Alfredo	1 entrée	240	5/2.5	2	na	na	na	na	na	0	na
Fettucini Alfredo, w/ chicken	1 entrée	280	7/2.5	4	na	na	na	na	na	2.4	na
Lasagna	1 entrée	280	6/2	5	na	na	na	na	na	3.6	na
Lasagna w/ meat	1 entrée	360	9/3	7	na	na	na	na	na	1.2	na
Macaroni and cheese	1 entrée	250	6/2.5	3	na	na	na	na	na	3	na
Manicotti with three cheeses	1 entrée	300	9/3	5	na	na	na	na	na	5	na
Pizza, cheese	1 pizza	340	5/1.5	5	na	na	na	na	na	0	na
Pizza, pepperoni	1 pizza	340	5/1.5	6	na	na	na	na	na	0	na
Pizza, supreme	1 pizza	330	5/1.5	6	na	na	na	na	na	0	na
Pizza, vegetable	1 pizza	280	4/1.5	5	na	na	na	na	na	0	na
Pork, country breaded w/ cheddar bacon potatoes	1 entrée	280	6/2.5	4	na	na	na	na	na	6	na
Ravioli, cheese	1 entrée	260	5/2.5	4	na	na	na	na	na	0	na
Rigatoni w/ broccoli and chicken	1 entrée	280	7/2.5	3	na	na	na	na	na	18	na
Salisbury steak w/ redskin mashed potatoes	1 entrée	210	6/2.5	3	na	na	na	na	na	5	na
Southwestern style rice and beans	1 entrée	250	3/1	5	na	na	na	na	na	0	na

118

Food	Serving Size	Calories	Fat/Sat. Fat (gm)	Fiber (gm)	Flavonoids (mg)	Carotenoids (mcg or mg)	PE (mcg or mg)	Folate (mcg)	Selenium (mcg)	Vit. C (mg)	Vit. E (IUs)
Spaghetti w/ meatballs	1 entrée	290	8/2.5	7	na	na	na	na	na	3.6	na
Tuna casserole	1 entrée	240	7/2	4	na	na	na	na	na	0	na
Turkey breast, roasted	1 entrée	220	5/2	5	na	na	na	na	na	1.2	na
Turkey, roasted w/ mashed potatoes	1 entrée	200	5/2	4	na	na	na	na	na	3.6	na
ENTRÉES/LEAN CUISINE											
Beef, Hunan beef and broccoli	1 entrée	240	3.5/1	2	na	na	na	na	na	6	na
Beef, oriental	1 entrée	210	3.5/1.5	2	na	na	na	na	na	3.6	na
Beef, oven roasted	1 entrée	240	8/3.5	3	na	na	na	na	na	3.6	na
Beef peppercorn	1 entrée	260	7/2	4	na	na	na	na	na	5	na
Beef portobello	1 entrée	220	7/3.5	2	na	na	na	na	na	0	na
Beef pot roast	1 entrée	190	6/2	3	na	na	na	na	na	0	na
Beef tips	1 entrée	270	6/2.5	4	na	na	na	na	na	3.6	na
Chicken, baked	1 entrée	240	4.5/1.5	3	na	na	na	na	na	0	na
Chicken and bow tie pasta	1 entrée	220	4/1	5	na	na	na	na	na	15	na
Chicken carbonara	1 entrée	260	8/2	2	na	na	na	na	na	5	na
Chicken chow mein	1 entrée	240	3.5/1	3	na	na	na	na	na	0	na
Chicken enchilada	1 entrée	280	5/1.5	3	na	na	na	na	na	2.4	na
Chicken, glazed	1 entrée	230	5/1	0	na	na	na	na	na	2.4	na
Chicken, grilled	1 entrée	250	5/1.5	3	na	na	na	na	na	**18**	na
Chicken, herb roasted	1 entrée	200	3.5/1	3	na	na	na	na	na	**21**	na

119

Food	Serving Size	Calories	Fat/Sat. Fat (gm)	Fiber (gm)	Flavonoids (mg)	Carotenoids (mcg or mg)	PE (mcg or mg)	Folate (mcg)	Selenium (mcg)	Vit. C (mg)	Vit. E (IUs)
Chicken l'orange	1 entrée	230	1.5/0.5	2	na	na	na	na	na	9	na
Chicken, Mandarin	1 entrée	240	4/1	2	na	na	na	na	na	6	na
Chicken Mediterranean	1 entrée	260	4/0.5	4	na	na	na	na	na	5	na
Chicken parmesan	1 entrée	300	6/2	5	na	na	na	na	na	9	na
Chicken piccata	1 entrée	300	9/2.5	2	na	na	na	na	na	12	na
Chicken, roasted	1 entrée	250	7/2	3	na	na	na	na	na	1.2	na
Chicken, sweet and sour	1 entrée	320	3/1	1	na	na	na	na	na	12	na
Chicken teriyaki	1 entrée	320	3.5/1.5	0	na	na	na	na	na	2.4	na
Chicken w/ vegetables	1 entrée	250	5/2.5	3	na	na	na	na	na	2.4	na
Chicken in wine sauce	1 entrée	220	5/2.5	2	na	na	na	na	na	1.2	na
Fettucini Alfredo	1 entrée	280	7/3.5	2	na	na	na	na	na	0	na
Fish, baked	1 entrée	290	6/3	2	na	na	na	na	na	9	na
Lasagna, cheese	1 entrée	240	4.5/2.5	5	na	na	na	na	na	5	na
Lasagna w/ chicken	1 entrée	280	7/3	2	na	na	na	na	na	2.4	na
Lasagna w/ chicken and cheese	1 entrée	270	8/2.5	3	na	na	na	na	na	9	na
Lasagna w/ meat sauce	1 entrée	300	8/4.5	4	na	na	na	na	na	6	na
Lasagna, vegetable	1 entrée	260	7/3.5	4	na	na	na	na	na	5	na
Macaroni and cheese	1 entrée	290	7/4	2	na	na	na	na	na	0	na
Meatloaf and whipped potatoes	1 entrée	260	7/4	4	na	na	na	na	na	0	na
Pizza, cheese	1 pizza	340	8/4	3	na	na	na	na	na	2.4	na
Pizza, deluxe	1 pizza	330	9/3.5	3	na	na	na	na	na	9	na

Food	Serving Size	Calories	Fat/Sat. Fat (gm)	Fiber (gm)	Flavonoids (mg)	Carotenoids (mcg or mg)	PE (mcg or mg)	Folate (mcg)	Selenium (mcg)	Vit. C (mg)	Vit. E (IUs)
Pizza, pepperoni	1 pizza	300	7/2.5	2	na	na	na	na	na	2.4	na
Pork, honey roasted	1 entrée	240	5/2	3	na	na	na	na	na	6	na
Ravioli, cheese	1 entrée	260	7/3.5	4	na	na	na	na	na	5	na
Salisbury steak	1 entrée	290	9/4.5	3	na	na	na	na	na	1.2	na
Santa Fe rice and beans	1 entrée	300	5/2	6	na	na	na	na	na	6	na
Shrimp and angel hair pasta	1 entrée	280	5/1	3	na	na	na	na	na	24	na
Spaghetti w/ meat sauce	1 entrée	300	5/1.5	6	na	na	na	na	na	5	na
Spaghetti w/ meatballs	1 entrée	270	6/2.5	4	na	na	na	na	na	6	na
Stuffed cabbage	1 entrée	210	8/3.5	5	na	na	na	na	na	3.6	na
Swedish meatballs	1 entrée	290	7/3	4	na	na	na	na	na	0	na
Three-bean chili	1 entrée	280	8/2.5	8	na	na	na	na	na	18	na
Turkey breast, roasted	1 entrée	270	2/0.5	3	na	na	na	na	na	54	na
Turkey, glazed tenderloins	1 entrée	260	4.5/1	4	na	na	na	na	na	0	na
ENTRÉES/LEAN CUISINE (SKILLET SENSATION ENTREES)											
Beef teriyaki w/ rice	1 entrée	290	4/1.5	6	na	na	na	na	na	12	na
Chicken Alfredo	1 entrée	320	7/3.5	4	na	na	na	na	na	24	na
Chicken, garlic	1 entrée	340	4.5/2	4	na	na	na	na	na	54	na
Chicken, herb roasted w/ potatoes	1 entrée	250	4/1	4	na	na	na	na	na	12	na
Chicken, oriental	1 entrée	280	4/1	5	na	na	na	na	na	12	na
Chicken primavera	1 entrée	300	4/1	5	na	na	na	na	na	18	na
Chicken teriyaki	1 entrée	310	3.5/1.5	6	na	na	na	na	na	15	na

Food	Serving Size	Calories	Fat/Sat. Fat (gm)	Fiber (gm)	Flavonoids (mg)	Carotenoids (mcg or mg)	PE (mcg or mg)	Folate (mcg)	Selenium (mcg)	Vit. C (mg)	Vit. E (IUs)
Chicken, three cheese	1 entrée	350	9/3.5	3	na	na	na	na	na	12	na
Turkey, roasted	1 entrée	220	2/0.5	6	na	na	na	na	na	**60**	na
ENTRÉES/MRS. PAUL'S											
Fish, Dijon light	1 entrée	200	5/2	0	na	na	na	na	na	na	na
Fish, fillet, Florentine	1 entrée	220	8/4	0	na	na	na	na	na	na	na
Fish, Mornay, light	1 entrée	230	10/4	0	na	na	na	na	na	na	na
ENTRÉES/WEIGHT WATCHERS											
Beef Cantonese	1 entrée	200	4/1	0	na	na	na	na	na	na	na
Beef and macaroni	1 entrée	220	4.5/1.5	4	na	na	na	na	na	12	na
Beef Romanoff	1 entrée	230	7/3	0	na	na	na	na	na	na	na
Beef stir fry	1 entrée	150	3/2	0	na	na	na	na	na	2.4	na
Chicken enchilada	1 entrée	270	9/4.5	4	na	na	na	na	na	6	na
Chicken fettuccini	1 entrée	290	7/2	4	na	na	na	na	na	1.2	na
Chicken, glazed barbecue	1 entrée	230	2.5/0.5	4	na	na	na	na	na	na	na
Chicken, Mexican	1 entrée	220	7/2	0	na	na	na	na	na	na	na
Chicken, orange	1 entrée	170	2/1	0	na	na	na	na	na	2.4	na
Chicken, parmigiana	1 entrée	310	7/2	4	na	na	na	na	na	**18**	na
Chicken, roasted	1 entrée	240	6/1	4	na	na	na	na	na	na	na
Lasagna	1 entrée	300	7/3	4	na	na	na	na	na	na	na
Macaroni and cheese	1 entrée	300	7/3	2	na	na	na	na	na	na	na
Pasta and mushrooms marsala	1 entrée	280	9/3.5	5	na	na	na	na	na	2.4	na

Food	Serving Size	Calories	Fat/Sat. Fat (gm)	Fiber (gm)	Flavonoids (mg)	Carotenoids (mcg or mg)	PE (mcg or mg)	Folate (mcg)	Selenium (mcg)	Vit. C (mg)	Vit. E (IUs)
Pasta and spinach Romano	1 entrée	240	8/3.5	4	na	na	na	na	na	9	na
Pasta, tomato basil	1 entrée	260	9/3.5	5	na	na	na	na	na	3.6	na
Pizza, cheese	6 oz.	300	7/2	0	na	na	na	na	na	na	na
Pizza, deluxe combination	1 serving	380	11/3.5	6	na	na	na	na	na	5	na
Pizza, extra cheese	1 serving	390	12/4	6	na	na	na	na	na	6	na
Pizza, pepperoni	1 serving	390	12/4	4	na	na	na	na	na	5	na
Ravioli, cheese	1 entrée	240	6/2	0	na	na	na	na	na	na	na
Salisbury steak	1 entrée	260	10/5	3	na	na	na	na	na	na	na
Turkey breast, stuffed	1 entrée	230	5/1	6	na	na	na	na	na	6	na
Ziti mozzarella pasta	1 entrée	280	6/1.5	4	na	na	na	na	na	na	na

ENTRÉES/VEGETARIAN ENTRÉES

Food	Serving Size	Calories	Fat/Sat. Fat (gm)	Fiber (gm)	Flavonoids (mg)	Carotenoids (mcg or mg)	PE (mcg or mg)	Folate (mcg)	Selenium (mcg)	Vit. C (mg)	Vit. E (IUs)
Bean loaf (Natural Touch)	1 slice	160	8/1.5	5	na	na	na	na	na	1.3	na
Black bean vegetable enchilada (Amy's Kitchen)	1 serving	130	4/0	2	na	na	na	na	na	na	na
Hearty Chik'n Vegetables Pot Pie, meatless (Morningstar Farms)	1 pie	350	14/3.5	9	na	na	na	na	na	0	na
Fried Chik'N w/ gravy, meatless (Loma Linda)	2 pieces	160	10/1.5	2	na	na	na	na	na	0	na
Lentil rice loaf (Natural Touch)	1 slice	160	7/1	4	na	na	na	na	na	0	na

123

Food	Serving Size	Calories	Fat/Sat. Fat (gm)	Fiber (gm)	Flavonoids (mg)	Carotenoids (mcg or mg)	PE (mcg or mg)	Folate (mcg)	Selenium (mcg)	Vit. C (mg)	Vit. E (IUs)
Macaroni and soy cheese (Amy's Kitchen)	1 serving	360	14/1	4	na	na	na	na	na	na	na
Salisbury steak, meatless (Amy's Kitchen)	1 entrée	420	16/5	9	na	na	na	na	na	na	na
Swiss steak, meatless (Loma Linda)	1 entrée	120	6/1	4	na	na	na	na	na	0	na
Thai stir fry w/ tofu and vegetables (Amy's Kitchen)	1 serving	270	11/7	2	na	na	na	na	na	na	na
Vegetable lasagna (Amy's Kitchen)	1 serving	280	12/4.5	3	na	na	na	na	na	na	na
Vegetable lasagna w/ tofu (Amy's Kitchen)	1 serving	300	10/1	6	na	na	na	na	na	na	na
FAST FOODS/BREAKFAST FOODS											
Burger King:											
Biscuit	1 biscuit	300	15/3.5	t	0	0	0	na	na	0	na
French Toast Sticks	5 sticks	390	20/4.5	2	0	0	0	na	na	0	na
Hardee's:											
Apple, Cinnamon & Raisin Biscuit	1 biscuit	250	8/2	na	0	0	0	na	na	na	na
Chicken Biscuit	1 biscuit	590	27/7	na	0	0	0	na	na	na	na

Food	Serving Size	Calories	Fat/Sat. Fat (gm)	Fiber (gm)	Flavonoids (mg)	Carotenoids (mcg or mg)	PE (mcg or mg)	Folate (mcg)	Selenium (mcg)	Vit. C (mg)	Vit. E (IUs)
Made from Scratch											
Biscuit	1 biscuit	390	21/6	na	0	0	0	na	na	na	na
Omelet Biscuit	1 biscuit	550	32/12	na	0	0	0	na	na	na	na
Jack in the Box:											
Breakfast Jack	1 serving	310	14/5	1	0	0	0	na	na	na	na
French Toast Sticks	4 sticks	430	18/4	2	0	0	0	na	na	na	na
Sourdough Breakfast Sandwich	1 serving	450	26/8	2	0	0	0	na	na	na	na
McDonald's:											
Biscuit	1 biscuit	240	11/2.5	1	0	0	0	na	na	0	na
Egg McMuffin	1 serving	290	12/4.5	1	0	0	0	na	na	1.2	na
Lowfat Apple Bran Muffin	1 muffin	300	3/0.5	3	0	0	0	na	na	0	na
Scrambled Eggs	2 eggs	160	11/3.5	0	0	0	0	na	na	0	na
Spanish Omelet Bagel	1 bagel	690	38/14	3	0	0	0	na	na	15	na
Subway:											
Ham & Egg Sandwich	1 sandwich	291	12/3	1	0	0	0	na	na	15	na
Western Egg Sandwich	1 sandwich	285	12/2.5	2	0	0	0	na	na	24	na
FAST FOODS/BURGERS											
Burger King:											
Whopper w/o mayo	1 burger	530	22/9	4	0	0	0	na	na	9	na
Hamburger	1 burger	320	14/6	2	0	0	0	na	na	0	na

125

Food	Serving Size	Calories	Fat/Sat Fat (gm)	Fiber (gm)	Flavonoids (mg)	Carotenoids (mcg or mg)	PE (mcg or mg)	Folate (mcg)	Selenium (mcg)	Vit. C (mg)	Vit. E (IUs)
Dairy Queen:											
DQ Homestyle Hamburger	1 burger	290	12/5	2	0	0	0	na	na	3.6	na
Hardee's:											
Hamburger	1 burger	270	11/4	na	0	0	0	na	na	na	na
Jack in the Box:											
Hamburger	1 burger	250	9/3.5	2	0	0	0	na	na	na	na
Sourdough Jack	1 serving	660	47/16	3	0	0	0	na	na	na	na
McDonald's:											
Hamburger	1 burger	280	10/4	2	0	0	0	na	na	2.4	na
Quarter Pounder	1 burger	430	21/8	2	0	0	0	na	na	2.4	na
Wendy's:											
Classic Single w/ Everything	1 burger	410	19/7	2	0	0	0	na	na	9	na
FAST FOODS/DESSERTS											
Dairy Queen:											
DQ Fudge Bar— sugar-free	1 bar	50	0/0	0	0	0	0	na	na	0	na
DQ Vanilla Orange Bar— sugar-free	1 bar	60	0/0	0	0	na	0	na	na	0	na
McDonald's:											
Fruit n' Yogurt Parfait	1 serving	380	5/2	2	0	0	0	na	na	24	na

Food	Serving Size	Calories	Fat/Sat. Fat (gm)	Fiber (gm)	Flavonoids (mg)	Carotenoids (mcg or mg)	PE (mcg or mg)	Folate (mg)	Selenium (mcg)	Vit. C (mg)	Vit. E (IUs)
Fruit n' Yogurt Parfait w/o granola	1 serving	280	4/2	t	0	0	0	na	na	**24**	na
Vanilla Reduced Fat Ice Cream Cone	1 serving	150	4.5/3	0	0	0	0	na	na	1.2	na
Wendy's:											
Frostie	1 small	330	8/5	0	0	0	0	na	na	0	na
FAST FOODS/MEXICAN FOODS											
Jack in the Box:											
Monster Taco	1 taco	280	17/6	3	na	na	0	na	na	na	na
Taco	1 taco	180	10/3.5	2	na	na	0	na	na	na	na
Taco Bell:											
Burrito, Bean	1 serving	370	12/3.5	**12**	na	na	na	na	na	na	na
Burrito, Chili Cheese	1 serving	330	13/5	4	na	na	na	na	na	na	na
Burrito, Double Supreme—Chicken	1 serving	460	17/6	3	na	na	na	na	na	na	na
Burrito, Fiesta—Chicken	1 serving	370	12/3.5	3	na	na	na	na	na	na	na
Burrito—7-Layer	1 serving	520	22/7	**13**	na	na	na	na	na	na	na
Burrito, Supreme—Chicken	1 serving	410	16/6	**8**	na	na	na	na	na	na	na
Chalupa Baja—Chicken	1 serving	400	24/5	2	na	na	na	na	na	na	na

127

Food	Serving Size	Calories	Fat/Sat. Fat (gm)	Fiber (gm)	Flavonoids (mg)	Carotenoids (mcg or mg)	PE (mcg or mg)	Folate (mcg)	Selenium (mcg)	Vit. C (mg)	Vit. E (IUs)
Chalupa Nacho Cheese—Chicken	1 serving	350	19/4.5	2	na	na	na	na	na	na	na
Chalupa Santa Fe—Chicken	1 serving	420	26/6	2	na	na	na	na	na	na	na
Chalupa Supreme—Chicken	1 serving	360	20/7	2	na	na	na	na	na	na	na
Enchirito, Chicken	1 serving	350	16/8	7	na	na	na	na	na	na	na
Gordita Baja—Chicken	1 serving	340	18/4	3	na	na	na	na	na	na	na
Gordita Nacho Cheese—Chicken	1 serving	290	13/2.5	3	na	na	na	na	na	na	na
Gordita Santa Fe—Chicken	1 serving	370	20/4	3	na	na	na	na	na	na	na
Gordita Supreme—Chicken	1 serving	300	13/5	3	na	na	na	na	na	na	na
Taco	1 taco	210	12/4	3	na	na	na	na	na	na	na
Taco, Double Decker	1 taco	380	17/5	9	na	na	na	na	na	na	na
Taco, Double Decker Supreme	1 taco	420	21/8	10	na	na	na	na	na	na	na
Taco, Soft—Chicken	1 taco	190	7/2.5	2	na	na	na	na	na	na	na
Taco Supreme	1 taco	260	16/6	4	na	na	na	na	na	na	na
Tostada	1 serving	250	12/4.5	11	na	na	na	na	na	na	na

Food	Serving Size	Calories	Fat/Sat Fat (gm)	Fiber (gm)	Flavonoids (mg)	Carotenoids (mcg or mg)	PE (mcg or mg)	Folate (mcg)	Selenium (mcg)	Vit. C (mg)	Vit. E (IUs)
FAST FOODS/PASTA											
Fazoli's:											
Baked Ravioli w/ Meat Sauce	1 serving	790	29/15	6	na	na	0	na	na	na	na
Baked Rigatoni	1 serving	470	18/8	4	na	na	0	na	na	na	na
Baked Ziti—Regular	1 serving	750	26/11	6	na	na	0	na	na	na	na
Broccoli Fettuccine Alfredo	1 serving	560	15/4	6	na	na	0	na	na	na	na
Broccoli Lasagna	1 serving	420	18/5	5	na	na	0	na	na	na	na
Lasagna	1 serving	440	19/6	4	na	na	0	na	na	na	na
Manicotti w/ Tomato Sauce	1 serving	290	15/8	2	na	na	0	na	na	na	na
Spaghetti w/ Tomato Sauce—regular	1 serving	620	8/1	7	na	na	0	na	na	na	na
Pizza Hut:											
Cavatini Pasta	1 serving	480	14/6	9	na	na	0	na	na	na	na
Spaghetti w/ Marinara	1 serving	490	6/1	8	na	na	0	na	na	na	na
Spaghetti w/ Meatballs	1 serving	850	24/10	10	na	na	0	na	na	na	na
FAST FOODS/PIZZA											
Fazoli's:											
Cheese Pizza	1 slice	460	15/8	2	na	na	0	na	na	na	na
Combination Pizza	1 slice	570	25/12	3	na	na	0	na	na	na	na

Food	Serving Size	Calories	Fat/Sat. Fat (gm)	Fiber (gm)	Flavonoids (mg)	Carotenoids (mcg or mg)	PE (mcg or mg)	Folate (mcg)	Selenium (mcg)	Vit. C (mg)	Vit. E (IUs)
Pizza Hut:											
Cheese	1 slice	240	10/5	2	0	0	0	na	na	2.4	na
Chicken Supreme	1 slice	230	7/3.5	2	0	0	0	na	na	6	na
Veggie Lover's	1 slice	220	8/3	2	na	na	na	na	na	9	na
FAST FOODS/POULTRY (INCLUDING CHICKEN SANDWICHES)											
Arby's:											
Chicken Breast Fillet Sandwich	1 serving	540	30/5	2	0	0	0	na	na	3.6	na
Chicken Cordon Bleu Sandwich	1 serving	630	35/8	2	0	0	0	na	na	2.4	na
Grilled Chicken Deluxe Sandwich	1 serving	450	22/4	2	0	0	0	na	na	1	na
Light Grilled Chicken Sandwich	1 serving	280	5/1.5	3	0	0	0	na	na	0	na
Light Roast Chicken Deluxe Sandwich	1 serving	260	5/0.5	3	0	0	0	na	na	1	na
Burger King:											
BK Broiler Chicken Sandwich	1 serving	550	25/5	3	0	0	0	na	na	6	na
Chicken Sandwich w/o mayo	1 serving	460	17/5	3	0	0	0	na	na	0	na

130

Food	Serving Size	Calories	Fat/Sat. Fat (gm)	Fiber (gm)	Flavonoids (mg)	Carotenoids (mcg or mg)	PE (mcg or mg)	Folate (mcg)	Selenium (mcg)	Vit. C (mg)	Vit. E (IUs)
Dairy Queen:											
Chicken Breast Fillet Sandwich	1 serving	430	20/4	2	0	0	0	na	na	0	na
Grilled Chicken Sandwich	1 serving	310	10/2.5	3	0	0	0	na	na	0	na
Hardee's:											
Breast	1 piece	370	15/4	na	0	0	0	na	na	na	na
Chicken Fillet Sandwich	1 serving	480	23/4	na	0	0	0	na	na	na	na
Grilled Chicken Sandwich	1 serving	350	16/3	na	0	0	0	na	na	na	na
Leg	1 piece	170	7/2	na	0	0	0	na	na	na	na
Jack in the Box:											
Chicken Breast Pieces	5 pieces	360	17/3	1	0	0	0	na	na	na	na
Chicken Fajita Pita	1 serving	330	11/4.5	3	0	0	0	na	na	na	na
Chicken Sandwich	1 serving	410	21/4.5	2	0	0	0	na	na	na	na
Chicken Supreme	1 serving	710	39/11	4	0	0	0	na	na	na	na
Chicken Teriyaki Bowl	1 serving	550	3/0.5	3	0	0	0	na	na	na	na
Grilled Chicken Fillet	1 serving	430	22/6	2	0	0	0	na	na	na	na
Jack's Spicy Chicken	1 serving	580	31/6	3	0	0	0	na	na	na	na
Fazoli's:											
Chicken Caesar Club Panini	1 serving	660	35/11	3	na	na	0	na	na	na	na
Chicken Pesto Panini	1 serving	510	20/6	3	na	na	0	na	na	na	na
Smoked Turkey Panini	1 serving	710	38/12	3	na	na	0	na	na	na	na

Food	Serving Size	Calories	Fat/Sat. Fat (gm)	Fiber (gm)	Flavonoids (mg)	Carotenoids (mcg or mg)	PE (mcg or mg)	Folate (mcg)	Selenium (mcg)	Vit. C (mg)	Vit. E (IUs)
Kentucky Fried Chicken:											
Hot & Spicy Chicken—Breast	1 piece	505	29/8	1	0	0	0	na	na	0	na
Original Recipe Chicken—Breast	1 piece	400	24/6	1	0	0	0	na	na	0	na
Original Recipe Sandwich w/o sauce	1 serving	360	13/3.5	t	0	0	0	na	na	0	na
Tender Roast Chicken Sandwich w/o sauce	1 serving	270	5/1.5	1	0	0	0	na	na	0	na
Long John Silver's:											
Chicken Sandwich	1 sandwich	340	14/3.5	na	0	0	0	na	na	na	na
McDonald's:											
Chicken McGrill w/o mayo	1 sandwich	340	7/1.5	2	0	0	0	na	na	6	na
Chicken McNuggets	6 pieces	290	17/3.5	2	0	0	0	na	na	0	na
Wendy's:											
Chicken Breast Fillet Sandwich	1 sandwich	430	16/3	2	0	0	0	na	na	12	na
Chicken Club Sandwich	1 sandwich	470	20/4.5	2	0	0	0	na	na	12	na
Crispy Chicken Nuggets	5 pieces	230	16/3	0	0	0	0	na	na	1.2	na
Grilled Chicken Sandwich	1 sandwich	300	7/1.5	2	0	0	0	na	na	9	na
Spicy Chicken Sandwich	1 sandwich	410	14/2.5	2	0	0	0	na	na	9	na

132

Food	Serving Size	Calories	Fat/Sat. Fat (gm)	Fiber (gm)	Flavonoids (mg)	Carotenoids (mcg or mg)	PE (mcg or mg)	Folate (mcg)	Selenium (mcg)	Vit. C (mg)	Vit. E (IUs)
FAST FOODS/SALADS*											
Arby's:											
Caesar Salad	1 serving	90	4/2.5	3	na	na	na	na	na	**42**	na
Caesar Side Salad	1 serving	45	2/1	2	na	na	na	na	na	**27**	na
Garden Salad	1 serving	70	1/0	6	na	na	na	na	na	**42**	na
Grilled Chicken Caesar Salad	1 serving	230	8/3.5	3	na	na	na	na	na	**42**	na
Grilled Chicken Salad	1 serving	210	4.5/1.5	6	na	na	na	na	na	**42**	na
Roast Chicken Salad	1 serving	160	2.5/0	6	na	na	na	na	na	**42**	na
Side Salad	1 serving	25	0/0	2	na	na	na	na	na	9	na
Turkey Club Salad	1 serving	350	21/10	3	na	na	na	na	na	**42**	na
Jack in the Box:											
Side Salad	1 serving	50	3/1.5	2	na	na	na	na	na	na	na
Fazoli's:											
Chicken & Pasta Caesar Salad	1 serving	370	13/3	3	na	na	na	na	na	na	na
Garden Salad	1 serving	30	0/0	2	na	na	na	na	na	na	na
Italian Chef Salad	1 serving	260	21/9	3	na	na	na	na	na	na	na
Pasta Salad w/ dressing	1 serving	600	26/7	5	na	na	na	na	na	na	na
Side Pasta Salad w/ dressing	1 serving	240	10/3	2	na	na	na	na	na	na	na

*Dressing not included except where noted

133

Food	Serving Size	Calories	Fat/Sat. Fat (gm)	Fiber (gm)	Flavonoids (mg)	Carotenoids (mcg or mg)	PE (mcg or mg)	Folate (mcg)	Selenium (mcg)	Vit. C (mg)	Vit. E (IUs)
Long John Silver's:											
Garden Salad	1 serving	45	0/0	na	na	na	na	na	na	na	na
Grilled Chicken Salad	1 serving	140	2.5/0.5	na	na	na	na	na	na	na	na
Ocean Chef Salad	1 serving	130	2/0	na	na	na	na	na	na	na	na
Side Salad	1 serving	20	0/0	na	na	na	na	na	na	na	na
McDonald's:											
Chef Salad	1 serving	150	8/3.5	2	na	na	na	na	na	15	na
Garden Salad	1 serving	100	6/3	2	na	na	na	na	na	15	na
Grilled Chicken Caesar Salad	1 serving	100	2.5/1.5	2	na	na	na	na	na	12	na
Quizno's:											
Tuscan Chicken Salad	1 serving	326	6.3/1	4	na	na	na	na	na	na	na
Subway Salads (Lower fat):											
Ham	1 serving	112	3/1	3	na	na	na	na	na	30	na
Roast Beef	1 serving	114	3/0.5	3	na	na	na	na	na	30	na
Roasted Chicken Breast	1 serving	137	3/0.5	3	na	na	na	na	na	30	na
Subway Club	1 serving	145	3.5/1	3	na	na	na	na	na	30	na
Tuna w/ light mayo	1 serving	238	16/4	3	na	na	na	na	na	30	na
Turkey Breast	1 serving	105	2/0.5	3	na	na	na	na	na	30	na
Turkey Breast & Ham	1 serving	117	3/0.5	3	na	na	na	na	na	30	na
Veggie Delite	1 serving	50	1/0	3	na	na	na	na	na	30	na

Food	Serving Size	Calories	Fat/Sat. Fat (gm)	Fiber (gm)	Flavonoids (mg)	Carotenoids (mcg or mg)	PE (mcg or mg)	Folate (mcg)	Selenium (mcg)	Vit. C (mg)	Vit. E (IUs)
Taco Bell:											
Taco Salad w/ Salsa	1 serving	850	52/14	16	na	na	na	na	na	na	na
Taco Salad w/ Salsa, no shell	1 serving	400	22/10	15	na	na	na	na	na	na	na
Wendy's:											
Caesar Side Salad	1 serving	110	5/2.5	1	na	na	na	na	na	15	na
Deluxe Garden Salad	1 serving	110	6/1	4	na	na	na	na	na	36	na
Grilled Chicken Salad	1 serving	200	7/1.5	4	na	na	na	na	na	36	na
Side Salad	1 serving	60	3/0.5	2	na	na	na	na	na	18	na
Taco Salad	1 serving	380	19/10	8	na	na	na	na	na	21	na

FAST FOODS/SANDWICHES (OTHER)

Food	Serving Size	Calories	Fat/Sat. Fat (gm)	Fiber (gm)	Flavonoids (mg)	Carotenoids (mcg or mg)	PE (mcg or mg)	Folate (mcg)	Selenium (mcg)	Vit. C (mg)	Vit. E (IUs)
Arby's:											
Arby-Q	1 serving	360	14/4	2	0	0	0	na	na	5	na
Regular Roast Beef	1 serving	350	16/6	2	0	0	0	na	na	0	na
Roast Chicken Caesar	1 serving	820	38/9	5	0	0	0	na	na	9	na
Roast Turkey & Swiss	1 serving	760	33/6	5	0	0	0	na	na	2.4	na
Hardee's:											
Big Roast Beef	1 serving	410	24/9	na	0	0	0	na	na	na	na
Regular Roast Beef	1 serving	310	16/6	na	0	0	0	na	na	na	na
Subway (Lower fat):											
Asiago Chicken Caesar Wrap	1 wrap	413	15/3	2	0	0	0	na	na	15	na

Food	Serving Size	Calories	Fat/Sat. Fat (gm)	Fiber (gm)	Flavonoids (mg)	Carotenoids (mcg or mg)	PE (mcg or mg)	Folate (mcg)	Selenium (mcg)	Vit. C (mg)	Vit. E (IUs)
Ham Deli	1 sandwich	194	3.5/1	2	0	0	0	na	na	24	na
Roast Beef Deli	1 sandwich	206	4/1	2	0	0	0	na	na	24	na
Turkey Breast Deli	1 sandwich	200	3.5/1	2	0	0	0	na	na	24	na

FAST FOODS/SEAFOOD (INCLUDING FISH SANDWICHES)

Food	Serving Size	Calories	Fat/Sat. Fat (gm)	Fiber (gm)	Flavonoids (mg)	Carotenoids (mcg or mg)	PE (mcg or mg)	Folate (mcg)	Selenium (mcg)	Vit. C (mg)	Vit. E (IUs)
Burger King:											
BK Big Fish Sandwich	1 sandwich	710	38/14	4	0	0	0	na	na	0	na
Hardee's:											
Fisherman's Fillet	1 sandwich	530	28/7	na	0	0	0	na	na	na	na
Long John Silver's:											
Breaded Clams	1 order	250	14/3.5	na	0	0	0	na	na	na	na
Country Style Breaded Fish	1 piece	200	10/1.5	na	0	0	0	na	na	na	na
Crabcake	1 crabcake	150	9/2	na	0	0	0	na	na	na	na
Flatbread Sandwich (Fish)	1 sandwich	740	48/9	na	0	0	0	na	na	na	na
Fish Sandwich	1 sandwich	430	20/5	na	0	0	0	na	na	na	na
Lemon Crumb Fish	2 pieces	240	12/4	na	0	0	0	na	na	na	na
Lemon Crumb Fish Meal	1 meal	730	29/6	na	na	na	0	na	na	na	na
Ultimate Fish Sandwich	1 sandwich	480	25/10	na	na	na	0	na	na	na	na
McDonald's:											
Filet-O-Fish	1 sandwich	470	26/5	1	0	0	0	na	na	na	na

Food	Serving Size	Calories	Fat/Sat. Fat (gm)	Fiber (gm)	Flavonoids (mg)	Carotenoids (mcg or mg)	PE (mcg or mg)	Folate (mcg)	Selenium (mcg)	Vit C (mg)	Vit E (IUs)
FAST FOODS/SIDES											
Arby's:											
Broccoli 'n Cheddar Baked Potato	1 potato	540	24/12	7	na	na	na	na	na	72	na
Deluxe Baked Potato	1 potato	650	34/20	6	na	na	na	na	na	36	na
Hardee's:											
Cole Slaw	1 serving	240	20/3	na	na	na	na	na	na	na	na
Mashed Potatoes	1 small serving	70	t/t	na	na	na	na	na	na	na	na
Kentucky Fried Chicken:											
BBQ Baked Beans	5½ oz.	190	3/1	6	na	na	na	na	na	na	na
Cole Slaw	5 oz.	232	13.5/2	3	na	na	na	na	na	na	na
Corn on the Cob	5.7 oz.	150	1.5/0	2	na	na	na	na	na	3.6	na
Green Beans	4.7 oz.	45	1.5/0.5	3	na	na	na	na	na	2.4	na
Mashed Potatoes w/ gravy	4.8 oz.	120	6/1	2	na	na	na	na	na	na	na
Mean Greens	5.4 oz.	70	3/1	5	na	na	na	na	na	6	na
Long John Silver's:											
Cole Slaw	4 oz.	170	7/0	na	na	na	na	na	na	na	na
Corn Cobbett	1 cobbette	80	0.5/0	na	na	na	na	na	na	na	na
Rice	4 oz.	180	4/0.5	na	na	na	na	na	na	na	na
Taco Bell:											
Mexican Rice	4¾ oz.	190	9/3.5	t	na	na	na	na	na	na	na

137

Food	Serving Size	Calories	Fat/Sat. Fat (gm)	Fiber (gm)	Flavonoids (mg)	Carotenoids (mcg or mg)	PE (mcg or mg)	Folate (mcg)	Selenium (mcg)	Vit. C (mg)	Vit. E (IUs)
Pinto Beans 'n Cheese	4½ oz.	180	8/4	10	na	na	na	na	na	na	na
Wendy's:											
Baked Potato, Broccoli & Cheese	10 oz.	470	14/3	9	na	na	na	na	na	72	na
Baked Potato, Plain	10 oz.	310	0/0	6	na	na	na	na	na	36	na
FAST FOODS/SOUP/CHILI											
Fazoli's:											
Minestrone Soup	1 serving	120	1/0	8	na	na	na	na	na	na	na
Long John Silver's:											
Clam Chowder	1 bowl	520	24/10	na	na	na	na	na	na	na	na
Subway:											
Black Bean	1 cup	180	4.5/2	15	na	na	na	na	na	5	na
Brown and Wild Rice w/ Chicken	1 cup	190	11/4.5	2	na	na	na	na	na	24	na
Chicken and Dumpling	1 cup	130	4.5/2.5	1	na	na	na	na	na	0	na
Cream of Potato w/ Bacon	1 cup	210	12/4	4	na	na	na	na	na	6	na
Golden Broccoli Cheese	1 cup	180	12/4	9	na	na	na	na	na	9	na
Minestrone	1 cup	70	1/0	0	na	na	na	na	na	6	na
New England Clam Chowder	1 cup	140	4.5/1	1	na	na	na	na	na	0	na
Potato Cheese Chowder	1 cup	210	10/7	2	na	na	na	na	na	0	na

138

Food	Serving Size	Calories	Fat/Sat. Fat (gm)	Fiber (gm)	Flavonoids (mg)	Carotenoids (mcg or mg)	PE (mcg or mg)	Folate (mcg)	Selenium (mcg)	Vit. C (mg)	Vit. E (IUs)
Roasted Chicken											
Noodle	1 cup	90	4/1	1	na	na	na	na	na	3.6	na
Tomato Bisque	1 cup	90	2.5/0.5	3	na	na	na	na	na	5	na
Vegetable Beef	1 cup	90	1.5/0.5	2	na	na	na	na	na	3.6	na
Wendy's:											
Chili, small	8 oz.	227	7/2.5	5	na	na	na	na	na	3.6	na
Chili, large	12 oz.	340	10/3.5	7	na	na	na	na	na	6	na

FAST FOODS/SUBS/GRINDERS/HOAGIES

Food	Serving Size	Calories	Fat/Sat. Fat (gm)	Fiber (gm)	Flavonoids (mg)	Carotenoids (mcg or mg)	PE (mcg or mg)	Folate (mcg)	Selenium (mcg)	Vit. C (mg)	Vit. E (IUs)
Arby's:											
French Dip	1 sub	440	18/8	2	0	0	0	na	na	1	na
Roast Beef	1 sub	760	48/16	3	0	0	0	na	na	3.6	na
Turkey	1 sub	630	37/9	2	0	0	0	na	na	2.4	na
Fazoli's:											
Submarino Original	1 sub	1160	55/17	8	na	na	na	na	na	na	na
Submarino Turkey	1 sub	990	34/10	7	0	0	0	na	na	na	na
Submarino Veggie	1 sub	1150	55/13	8	na	na	na	na	na	na	na
Quizno's:											
Honey Bourbon Sub	1 small sub	329	6/1	3	0	0	0	na	na	na	na
Turkey Lite Sub	1 small sub	334	6/1	3	0	0	0	na	na	na	na
Veggie Lite	1 small sub	300	6/1	5	na	na	na	na	na	na	na
Subway (Lowfat):											
Ham	1 6" sub	261	4.5/1.5	3	0	0	0	na	na	24	na

Food	Serving Size	Calories	Fat/Sat. Fat (gm)	Fiber (gm)	Flavonoids (mg)	Carotenoids (mcg or mg)	PE (mcg or mg)	Folate (mcg)	Selenium (mcg)	Vit. C (mg)	Vit. E (IUs)
Honey Mustard Turkey w/ Cucumber	16" sub	275	3.5/1	2	0	0	0	na	na	24	na
Roast Beef	16" sub	264	4.5/1	3	0	0	0	na	na	24	na
Roasted Chicken Breast	16" sub	311	6/1.5	3	0	0	0	na	na	24	na
Subway Club	16" sub	294	5/1.5	3	0	0	0	na	na	24	na
Turkey Breast	16" sub	254	3.5/1	3	0	0	0	na	na	24	na
Turkey Breast & Ham	16" sub	267	4.5/1	3	0	0	0	na	na	24	na
Veggie Delite	16" sub	200	2.5/0.5	3	na	na	0	na	na	24	na
FATS & OILS											
Beef tallow	1 tbsp.	115	13/6	0	0	0	0	0	0.03	0	0.5
Butter:											
Stick	1 pat	36	4/2.5	0	0	24 mcg (BC)	0	0.2	0.1	0	0.15
Whipped, stick	1 pat	27	3/2	0	0	19 mcg (BC)	0	0.1	0	0	0.15
Whipped, tub	1 tbsp.	67	7.6/4.7	0	0	47 mcg (BC)	0	0.3	0.1	0	0.15
Butter, light:											
Stick	1 pat	25	2.8/1.7	0	0	58 mcg (BC)	0	0.1	0.1	0	0.15
Whipped, tub	1 tbsp.	47	5/3.3	0	0	110 mcg (BC)	0	0.1	0.1	0	0.15
Butter-margarine blend:											
Stick	1 pat	36	4/1.7	0	0	33 mcg (BC)	na	0.1	0	0	0.5
Tub	1 tbsp.	102	11.5/4	0	0	117 mcg (BC)	na	0.3	0.1	0	1.5
Butter replacement, powdered:											
Molly McButter	1 tbsp.	23	0.1/0	0	0	0	0	0	0	0	0

Food	Serving Size	Calories	Fat/Sat. Fat (gm)	Fiber (gm)	Flavonoids (mg)	Carotenoids (mcg or mg)	PE (mcg or mg)	Folate (mcg)	Selenium (mcg)	Vit. C (mg)	Vit. E (IUs)
Lard	1 tbsp.	115	13/5	0	0	0	0	0	0.3	0	0.2
Margarine:											
Corn, hard	1 pat	34	3.7/0.7	0	0	na	na	0.06	0	0.008	1
Corn & Soybean	1 pat	34	3.7/0.7	0	0	na	na	0.06	0	0.008	na
Liquid, soybean	1 tbsp.	102	11/1	0	0	na	na	0.4	0	0.05	1
Lower calorie (Imperial)	1 tbsp.	50	6/1	0	0	na	na	na	na	na	na
Nonfat	1 tbsp.	5	0.2/0	0	0	0	na	0	0	0	0
Soybean, hard	1 pat	34	3.8/0.6	0	0	na	na	0.05	0	0.008	na
Soybean, soft	1 tbsp.	100	11/2.4	0	0	na	na	0.15	0	0.02	na
Spread, extra light (Weight Watchers)	1 tbsp.	50	6/1	0	0	na	na	na	na	na	na
Stick, regular	1 pat	27	3/0.5	0	0	41 mcg (BC)	na	0.1	0	0	0.75
Super light (Smart Beat)	1 tbsp.	20	2/0	0	0	na	na	na	na	0.6	na
Tub	1 tbsp.	102	11/2	0	0	117 mcg (BC)	na	0.1	0	0	2.5
Whipped, tub	1 tbsp.	67	7.6/1.2	0	0	77 mcg (BC)	na	0.1	0	0	1.5
Margarine-like spread:											
40% fat	1 tbsp.	50	5.6/0.9	0	0	na	na	0.1	0	0.015	na
60% fat	1 tbsp.	78	9/2	0	0	na	na	0.12	0	0.015	na
Shortening (Crisco)	1 tbsp.	110	12/3	0	0	0	na	na	na	0.6	na
Vegetable oil spreads:											
I Can't Believe It's Not Butter	1 tbsp.	90	10/2	0	0	118 mcg	na	na	na	na	na
Promise	1 tbsp.	35	4/0	0	0	118 mcg	na	na	na	na	na

Food	Serving Size	Calories	Fat/Sat. Fat (gm)	Fiber (gm)	Flavonoids (mg)	Carotenoids (mcg or mg)	PE (mcg or mg)	Folate (mcg)	Selenium (mcg)	Vit. C (mg)	Vit. E (IUs)
Squeezable	1 tbsp.	80	9/1.5	0	0	na	na	na	na	na	na
Oils:											
Canola	1 tbsp.	122	13.6/1	0	na	na	na	na	na	na	na
Corn	1 tbsp.	120	14/2	0	na	na	na	na	na	0	na
Flaxseed*	1 tbsp.	120	13.6/1.3	0	na	0	na	0	0	0	3.6
Grapeseed	1 tbsp.	120	13.6/1.3	0	na	na	na	na	na	0	na
Olive	1 tbsp.	120	14/0	0	na	na	na	na	na	0	na
Peanut	1 tbsp.	122	13.6/2.5	0	na	na	na	na	na	0	na
Popcorn	1 tbsp.	120	14/2	0	na	na	na	na	na	na	na
Safflower, linoleic over 70%	1 tbsp.	120	13.6/0.8	0	na	na	na	0	0	0	9
Soybean	1 tbsp.	122	13.6/2	0	na	na	na	0	0	0	4
Sunflower	1 tbsp.	120	13.6/1.4	0	na	na	na	0	0	0	11
Vegetable	1 tbsp.	122	13.6/2	0	na	na	na	na	0	0	0
Wheat germ	1 tbsp.	120	13.6/2.5	0	na	na	na	0	0	0	39
FISH & SHELLFISH											
Anchovy, canned in olive oil	6 fillets	25	1.5/0	0	0	0	0	na	10	na	na
Bass, baked or broiled	1 fillet	90	3/0.6	0	0	0	0	12	10	1.5	0
Bluefish	3 oz.	135	4.6/1	0	0	0	0	1.7	40	0	na
Catfish, breaded, fried	3 oz.	195	11/3	0	0	0	0	25.5	12	0	na

*Available in high-lignan formulations

Food	Serving Size	Calories	Fat/Sat. Fat (gm)	Fiber (gm)	Flavonoids (mg)	Carotenoids (mcg or mg)	PE (mcg or mg)	Folate (mcg)	Selenium (mcg)	Vit. C (mg)	Vit. E (IUs)
Catfish, cooked	3 oz.	129	7/1.5	0	0	0	0	6	12	0.8	na
Clams, canned	¼ cup	50	1.5/0.5	0	0	0	0	0	12	0	0
Clams, cooked	20 clams	281	3.7/0.19	0	0	0	0	55	122	42	0
Cod, Atlantic, cooked	3 oz.	89	0.7/0.14	0	0	0	0	7	32	0.85	0.25
Crab cake	1 cake	93	4.5/0.9	0	0	0	0	32	24	1.7	0
Crab, Alaska King, cooked	3 oz.	82	1.3/0.1	0	0	0	0	43	34	6.5	0
Crab, blue, canned	1 can (6½ oz.)	124	1.5/0.3	0	0	0	0	53	40	3.4	2
Crab, imitation	½ cup	80	1/0	0	0	0	0	0	0	0	0
Fish, packaged:											
Breaded, frozen (Van de Kamp's)	2 pieces	280	18/3	0	0	0	0	na	na	na	na
Sticks, breaded, frozen (Van de Kamp's)	4 pieces	200	12/2	0	0	0	0	na	na	na	na
Flounder, frozen, cooked	3 oz.	88	1.7/0	0	0	0	0	na	33	na	na
Grouper, cooked	3 oz.	100	1/0.25	0	0	0	0	8.6	40	0	na
Haddock, cooked	3 oz.	95	0.8/0.14	0	0	0	0	11	34	0	1.5
Halibut, cooked	3 oz.	119	2.5/0.35	0	0	0	0	12	40	0	2
Herring, pickled	1 cup	367	25/3	0	0	0	0	3.3	82	0	2
Lobster meat	1 cup	142	1/0.15	0	0	0	0	16	62	0	na
Mackerel, cooked	3 oz.	223	15/3.5	0	0	0	0	1.3	44	0.34	na
Mahi Mahi (Peter Pan Seafoods)	3½ oz. fillets	85	0.7/0	0	0	0	0	na	40	na	na

Food	Serving Size	Calories	Fat/Sat Fat (gm)	Fiber (gm)	Flavonoids (mg)	Carotenoids (mcg or mg)	PE (mcg or mg)	Folate (mcg)	Selenium (mcg)	Vit C (mg)	Vit E (IUs)
Ocean perch, cooked	3 oz.	103	1.8/0.3	0	0	0	0	9	47	0.7	na
Orange roughy	3 oz.	76	0.8/0.02	0	0	0	0	7	40	0	na
Oysters:											
Breaded, fried	6 medium	173	11/3	na	0	0	0	28	58.5	3.3	na
Canned, smoked, cottonseed oil (Reese)	1 can	170	9/4	0	0	0	0	na	66	na	na
Raw	6 medium	50	1.3/0.4	0	0	0	0	15	53.5	4	na
Steamed	6 medium	47	1.3/0.4	0	0	0	0	14	46	3.5	na
Pollock, cooked	1 fillet	68	0.7/0.1	0	0	0	0	2	26	0	0.15
Salmon:											
Cooked	3 oz.	175	11/2	0	0	31 mcg (BC)	0	29	35	3	2
Pink, Atlantic, canned	3½ qz.	140	6/2	0	0	0	0	12	29	0	2
Smoked	3 oz.	120	6/2	0	0	0	0	2	28	0	1.7
Sardines:											
Canned in mustard sauce (Underwood)	3¾ oz.	220	16/0	0	0	0	0	na	na	na	na
Canned in oil	3 oz.	240	20/0	0	0	0	0	na	na	na	na
Canned in tomato sauce (Underwood)	3¾ oz.	220	16/0	0	t	t	0	na	na	na	na
Canned in water	3 oz.	230	18/0	0	0	0	0	na	na	na	na
Scallops:											
Baked or broiled	1 cup	253	7.5/1.3	0	0	0	0	35	51	6.5	5
Floured or breaded	1 cup	292	15/3	0.4	0	0	0	30	36	3	4.5

Food	Serving Size	Calories	Fat/Sat. Fat (gm)	Fiber (gm)	Flavonoids (mg)	Carotenoids (mcg or mg)	PE (mcg or mg)	Folate (mcg)	Selenium (mcg)	Vit. C (mg)	Vit. E (IUs)
Shrimp:											
Breaded, fried	4 large	73	4/0.6	0.11	0	0	0	2.4	12.5	0.5	na
Butterfly, frozen (Gorton's)	4 oz.	160	1/0	0	0	0	0	na	na	na	na
Canned	10 shrimp	38	0.6/0.1	0	0	0	0	0.6	13	0.7	0.5
Steamed	4 large	22	0.2/0.06	0	0	0	0	0.7	9	0.5	0.17
Snapper, cooked	1 fillet	218	3/0.6	0	0	0	0	10	83	3	na
Sole, frozen, cooked (Gorton's)	5 oz.	110	1/0	0	0	0	0	na	na	na	na
Squid, fried	3 oz.	149	6/1.5	0	0	0	0	12	44	3.5	na
Surimi	3 oz.	84	0.8/0.15	0	0	0	0	1.4	24	0	na
Swordfish, baked	1 piece	164	5.5/1.5	0	0	0	0	2.4	64	1.2	na
Trout	1 fillet	118	5/1	0	0	0	0	9	10	0.3	na
Tuna:											
Canned in oil, light	3 oz.	167	9/1.5	0	0	0	0	na	65	0	na
Canned in water, light	3 oz.	106	2/0	0	0	0	0	na	68	na	na
Canned in water, white	3 oz.	123	2/0	0	0	0	0	na	68	na	na
Steak (SeaPak)	6 oz.	180	2/0	0	0	0	0	na	73	na	na
FLOUR & GRAINS/FLOURS											
Barley flour	1 cup	457	0.13/0.02	4.4	na	na	na	9	na	0	na
Bisquick	½ cup	240	8/2	0	na	na	na	na	na	na	na
Blue corn flour	1 cup	520	6/0	12	na	na	na	na	na	0	na

145

Food	Serving Size	Calories	Fat/Sat. Fat (gm)	Fiber (gm)	Flavonoids (mg)	Carotenoids (mcg or mg)	PE (mcg or mg)	Folate (mcg)	Selenium (mcg)	Vit. C (mg)	Vit. E (IUs)
Brown rice flour	1 cup	574	4.4/0.9	7	na	0	na	25	na	0	1.7
Buckwheat flour	1 cup	402	3.7/0.8	12	na	na	na	65	7	0	1.8
Carob flour	1 cup	229	0.7/0.09	41	na	6 mcg (BC)	na	30	5.5	0.2	1
Chick pea flour	1 cup	339	6/0.6	10	na	na	36 mg	402	59	0	na
Corn flour, masa	1 cup	416	4/0.6	11	na	na	•	213	17	0	0.4
Corn flour, white, whole grain	1 cup	422	4.6/0.6	11	na	na	na	29	18	0	0.4
Corn flour, yellow, whole grain	1 cup	422	4.5/0.6	16	na	na	na	29	18	0	0.4
Graham flour	1 cup	360	20/0	16	na	na	na	na	na	na	na
Kamut flour	1 cup	440	0/0	16	na	na	na	na	na	na	na
Oat flour	1 cup	400	8/0	t	na	na	na	na	na	0	na
Peanut flour, defatted	1 cup	196	0.3/0.03	9.5	na	na	na	149	4	0	0.04
Peanut flour, lowfat	1 cup	257	13/2	9.5	na	na	na	80	4	0	na
Potato flour	1 cup	571	0.5/0.15	9	na	na	na	25	1	4	0.4
Rye flour, dark	1 cup	415	3.5/0.4	29	na	na	na	77	46	0	5
Rye flour, light	1 cup	374	1.4/0.14	15	na	na	na	22	36	0	0.85
Rye flour, medium	1 cup	361	1.8/0.2	15	na	na	na	19	36	0	2
Spelt flour	1 cup	440	4/0	8	na	na	na	na	na	0	na
Sunflower seed flour	1 cup	209	1/0.08	3	na	na	na	142	37	0.8	1.5
Triticale flour	1 cup	439	2.4/0.4	19	na	0	na	96	0	0	4
White flour, all-purpose, enriched	1 cup	455	1/0.2	3.4	na	0	na	192.5	42	0	0.1

Food	Serving Size	Calories	Fat/Sat. Fat (gm)	Fiber (gm)	Flavonoids (mg)	Carotenoids (mcg or mg)	PE (mcg or mg)	Folate (mcg)	Selenium (mcg)	Vit. C (mg)	Vit. E (IUs)
White flour, cake	1 cup	496	1/0.2	2.4	na	0	na	211	7	0	0.1
White flour, self-rising, enriched	1 cup	442	1/0.2	3.4	na	0	na	192.5	43	0	0.1
White flour, tortilla	1 cup	450	12/4.5	na	na	na	na	151	na	0	na
White flour, unbleached	1 cup	455	1/0.2	3.4	na	0	na	192.5	42	0	0.7
White rice flour	1 cup	578	2/0.6	4	na	0	na	6	24	0	0.3
Whole wheat flour	1 cup	407	2/0.4	15	na	0	na	53	85	0	2.2
FLOUR & GRAINS/GRAINS											
Barley, pearled, cooked	1 cup	193	0.7/0.15	6	na	7 mcg (BC)	na	25	13.5	0	0.1
Basmati rice, cooked	1 cup	230	4/0	0	na	0	na	na	na	na	na
Brown rice, instant (Minute Rice)	1 cup	240	2/0	0	na	0	na	na	na	na	na
Brown rice, long-grain, cooked	1 cup	216	2/0.35	3.5	na	0	na	8	19	0	2
Brown rice, medium-grain, cooked	1 cup	218	1.6/0.3	3.5	na	0	na	8	na	0	na
Brown rice, short-grain, cooked	1 cup					0					
Brown rice, Spanish, cooked	1 cup	260	2.5/0.5	5	na	na	na	na	na	0.6	na
Bulgur, cooked	1 cup	151	0.4/0.07	8	na	0	na	33	1	0	0.08
Corn bran	1 cup	170	0.7/0.1	65	na	na	na	3	12.5	0	2.6

Food	Serving Size	Calories	Fat/Sat. Fat (gm)	Fiber (gm)	Flavonoids (mg)	Carotenoids (mcg or mg)	PE (mcg or mg)	Folate (mcg)	Selenium (mcg)	Vit. C (mg)	Vit. E (IUs)
Couscous, cooked	1 cup	176	0.25/0.05	2	na	na	na	23.5	43	na	0.03
Couscous pilaf mix, cooked	1 cup	196	0/0	0	na	na	na	na	na	na	na
Millet, cooked	1 cup	207	2/0.3	2	na	0	na	33	1.6	0	0.47
Quinoa	1 cup	636	10/1	10	na	na	na	83	na	0	na
Rice, chicken flavored (Rice-A-Roni)	⅓ cup	181	5/0.5	0.5	na	na	na	na	na	0	na
Rice, fried (La Choy)	1 cup	236	1/0.2	2	na	na	na	na	0	0	na
Rice, herb & butter (Rice-A-Roni)	⅓ cup	175	5/0.85	0.6	na	na	na	na	na	0.7	na
Rice, long-grain & wild (Rice-A-Roni)	⅓ cup	164	5/0.85	1.7	na	na	na	na	na	0.7	na
Rice pilaf (Rice-A-Roni)	⅓ cup	175	5/0.6	0.6	na	na	na	na	na	0	na
Rye	1 cup	566	4/0.5	25	na	na	na	101	60	0	4.8
Semolina	1 cup	601	1.75/0.25	6.5	na	na	na	257	149	0	0.15
Wheat bran (Hodgson Mill)	¼ cup	30	0/0	7	na	0	na	na	na	0	na
Wheat germ (Kretschmer)	2 tbsp.	50	1/0	2	na	0	na	na	na	0	na
Wheat:											
Hard red	1 cup	632	4/0.6	23	na	0	na	82.5	136	0	4
Hard white	1 cup	657	3/0.5	na	na	0	na	72	na	0	na
Soft red	1 cup	556	2.6/0.5	21	na	0	na	69	na	0	3.6
Soft white	1 cup	571	3/0.6	21	na	0	na	68	na	0	3.6
Sprouted	1 cup	214	1.4/0.2	1	na	0	na	41	46	3	0.08
White rice, instant, cooked	1 cup	162	0.3/0.1	1	na	0	na	68	7	0	0.15

Food	Serving Size	Calories	Fat/Sat. Fat (gm)	Fiber (gm)	Flavonoids (mg)	Carotenoids (mcg or mg)	PE (mcg or mg)	Folate (mcg)	Selenium (mcg)	Vit. C (mg)	Vit. E (IUs)
White rice, long-grain, cooked (Uncle Ben's)	1 cup	180	2/0	0	na	0	na	na	na	na	na
White rice, medium-grain, cooked	1 cup	242	0.4/0.1	0.6	na	0	na	108	14	0	na
White rice, short-grain, cooked	1 cup	242	0.35/0.09	na	na	0	na	110	14	0	na
White rice, Spanish or Mexican	1 cup	216	4/0.6	3	na	689 mcg (BC)	na	61	9.5	37	2
Wild rice, cooked	1 cup	166	0.6/0.08	3	na	0	na	43	1.3	0	0.6
FRUITS											
Acerola cherries, raw	1 cup	31.4	0.3/0.1	1.1	na	453 mcg (BC)	na	13.7	0.6	1,644	0.15
Apple: Raw (3/4" diameter), w/ skin	1 fruit	81	0.5/0.1	4	139–526	41 mcg (AC) 41 mcg (BC)	17 mcg (D)	4	0.4	8	0.6
Raw (3/4" diameter), w/o skin	1 fruit	63	0.34/t	2	na	na	na	0	t	4.4	t
Dried	5 pieces	78	0.1/t	3	na	na	na	0	t	1.2	t
Applesauce, sweetened	1 cup	194	0.5/0.1	3	na	16 mcg (BC)	na	1.5	0.8	4.3	0
Applesauce, unsweetened	1 cup	105	0.1/0	3	na	44 mcg (BC)	na	1.5	0.7	3	0
Apricots: Raw	1 fruit	17	0.14/0	0.9	na	894 mcg (BC)	na	3	t	3.5	t
Canned, heavy syrup	1 cup	214	0.21/0	4	na	2 mg (BC)	na	5	t	8	3.5

149

Food	Serving Size	Calories	Fat/Sat. Fat (gm)	Fiber (gm)	Flavonoids (mg)	Carotenoids (mcg or mg)	PE (mcg or mg)	Folate (mcg)	Selenium (mcg)	Vit. C (mg)	Vit. E (IUs)
Canned, juice pack	1 cup	117	0.1/0	4	na	2.5 mg(BC)	na	4	0.7	12	3
Canned, light syrup	1 cup	159	0.1/0	4	na	2 mg (BC)	na	4.3	0.8	6.8	3.5
Canned, water pack	1 cup	66	0.4/0	4	na	1.5 mg (BC)	na	4	0.7	8.3	3
Dried	10 halves	83	0.16/0	3	na	1.5 mg (BC)	1.5 mcg	4	t	t	t
Avocado, California	1 avocado.	278	26.5/4.2	8.7	204	633 mcg (BC)	133 mcg (L)	107	0.7	13.7	3.5
Avocado, Florida	1 avocado.	489	46.6/7.4	15	na	1.1 mg (BC)	133 mcg (L)	188	1.2	24	6
Banana (8" long)	1 fruit	109	0.57/0.2	3	163	56 mcg (BC)	0	22.5	1.3	11	t
Banana chips, dried	10 chips	51	0.9/0.7	0.9	na	23 mcg (BC)	0	1.7	0.5	0.9	0
Blackberries, raw	1 cup	75	0.56/0	7.6	na	138 mcg (BC)	5.35 mg (L)	49	1	30	1.5
Blueberries:											
Raw	1 cup	81	0.55/0	4	362	87 mcg (BC)	1.2 mg (L)	9	1	19	2
Frozen, sweetened	1 cup	186	0.3/0	5	na	55 mcg (BC)	na	16	1.4	2.3	2.4
Frozen, unsweetened	1 cup	79	1/0	4.2	na	46 mcg (AC) 74 mcg (BC)	na	10.4	0.9	4	2.4
Cherries, raw	10 cherries	49	0/0	1.5	47.6	518 mcg (BC)	na	3	t	5	t
Cherries, water pack	1 cup	114	0.3/0.1	2.7	462	238 mcg (BC)	na	10	0.7	5.5	t
Cranberries, raw	1 cup	46	0.2/0	4	186	29 mcg (BC)	4 mcg (D/G) 1 mg (L)	1.6	0.6	13	0.15
Currants, black	1 cup	123	t/0	5.4	na	80 mcg (BC)	225 mcg (D/G)0 165 mcg (L)	0	0	456	0
Currants, red	1 cup	67	t/0	4.5	na	80 mcg (BC)	na	0	0	55	0
Dates, whole without pits	5 dates	114	0.19/t	3	na	14 mcg (BC)	3 mcg (D/G)	5	t	0	t

Food	Serving Size	Calories	Fat/Sat. Fat (gm)	Fiber (gm)	Flavonoids (mg)	Carotenoids (mcg or mg)	PE (mcg or mg)	Folate (mcg)	Selenium (mcg)	Vit. C (mg)	Vit. E (IUs)
Dates, chopped	1 cup	490	1/t	13	na	na	na	22	t	0	t
Figs, dried	2 figs	97	0.44/0	3.6	na	30 mcg (BC)	2.3 mcg (D/G)	3	0.4	0.4	0
Figs, canned, light syrup	1 cup	174	0.3/0.1	4.5	na	60 mcg (BC)	na	5	1	2.5	3
Fruit cocktail, heavy syrup	1 cup	181	0.17/0	2.5	na	298 mcg (BC)	t	7	1.2	5	5
Fruit cocktail, juice pack	1 cup	109	0.02/0	2.4	na	441 mcg (BC)	na	6	1.2	6.4	0.75
Fruit cocktail, light syrup	1 cup	140	0.2/0	2.4	na	305 mcg (BC)	na	6.5	1.2	4.6	1
Fruit cocktail, water pack	1 cup	39.4	0.1/0	1.2	na	185 mcg (BC)	na	3.3	0.6	2.6	0.6
Grapefruit: Pink (¾" diameter)	1 half	37	0.12/0	1.3	28	741 mcg (BC) 1.8 mg (LYC)	na	15	1.7	47	0.5
White (3¾" diameter)	1 half	39	0.12/0	1.3	28	741 mcg (BC) 1.8 mg (LYC)	na	15	1.7	47	0.5
Canned sections, light syrup	1 cup	152	0.25/0	1	na	0	na	23	2.3	54	1
Canned sections, water pack	1 cup	88	0.2/0	1	na	0	na	21.5	2.2	53	1
Grapes, red	1 cup	114	0.93/0.3	1.6	592	67 mcg (BC)	na	6	0.3	17	1.5
Grapes, white	1 cup	114	0.93/0.3	1.6	310	67 mcg (BC)	na	6	0.3	17	1.5
Guava	1 medium	46	0.5/0.2	5	2,796	427 mcg (BC)	700 mcg (L)	12.6	0.5	165	1.5
Kiwi fruit, raw	1 fruit	46	2.6/0	2.6	na	82 mcg (BC)	2.3 mg (L)	29	0.5	75	1.4
Lemon, raw, without peel	1 fruit	17	1.6/0	1.6	24	10 mcg (BC)	36 mcg (L)	6	0.2	31	0.15

151

Food	Serving Size	Calories	Fat/Sat. Fat (gm)	Fiber (gm)	Flavonoids (mg)	Carotenoids (mcg or mg)	PE (mcg or mg)	Folate (mcg)	Selenium (mcg)	Vit. C (mg)	Vit. E (IUs)
Mango, diced	1 cup	107	0.45/0.1	3	69	3.8 mg (BC)	12 mcg (D/G)	23	1	46	3
Melons:											
Cantaloupe	½ melon	24	0.19/0	0.55	18	1.3 mg (BC)	127 mcg (L)	12	0.3	29	0.15
Casaba	1 cup	44	0.2/0	1.4	na	31 mcg (BC)	na	29	0.5	27	0.5
Honeydew	½ melon	56	0.2/0	1	61	38 mcg (BC)	5 mcg (D/G)	10	0.6	40	0.3
Nectarine (2½" diameter)	1 fruit	67	0.63/0.1	2	na	604 mcg (BC)	na	5	0.5	7.3	2
Orange, medium	1 fruit	62	0.16/0	3	54–251	165 mcg (BC) 160 mcg (BCR) 245 mcg (LU+Z)	101 mcg (L)	39	0.7	70	0.5
Orange sections, canned, juice pack	1 cup	93	0.3/0	3.4	na	236 mcg (BC)	na	41	0.7	92	0.6
Orange sections, raw	1 cup	85	0.22/0	4	na	na	na	54	1	96	t
Papaya, diced	1 cup	55	0.2/t	2.5	85	386 mcg (BC) 1 mg (BCR)	0	53	0.8	87	2.4
Papaya, whole	1 fruit	119	0.43/t	5.5	na	510 mcg (BC)	0	116	1.8	188	5
Passion fruit	1 fruit	18	0.1/0	2	na	76 mcg (BC)	17 mcg (D/G)	2.5	0.1	5.4	0.3
Peaches:											
Raw, medium	1 fruit	42	0.09/0	2	69	317 mcg (BC)	na	3	0.4	6.5	1
Canned, heavy syrup	1 cup	194	0.26/t	3.4	na	875 mcg (BC)	4 mcg (D/G)	8	t	7	3.5
Canned, juice pack	1 cup	109	0.07/0	3	na	570 mcg (BC)	na	7	0.8	9	5.5
Canned, water pack	1 cup	59	0.1/0	3	na	776 mcg (BC)	na	8	0.7	7	3.3
Dried	3 halves	96	0.3/0	3	na	518 mcg (BC)	na	0.1	0.9	2	0

Food	Serving Size	Calories	Fat/Sat. Fat (gm)	Fiber (gm)	Flavonoids (mg)	Carotenoids (mcg or mg)	PE (mcg or mg)	Folate (mcg)	Selenium (mcg)	Vit. C (mg)	Vit. E (IUs)
Frozen, sliced, sweetened	1 cup	235	0.3/0	4.5	na	420 mcg (BC)	na	8	1	235	3.3
Frozen, sliced, unsweetened	1 cup	107	0.2/0	5	na	767 mcg (BC)	na	8	1	236	2.5
Pears:											
Raw, medium	1 fruit	98	0.66/0	4	317	45 mcg (BC)	na	12	1.7	6.6	1
Canned, heavy syrup	1 cup	197	0.35/0	4	na	3 mcg (BC)	t	3	1.1	3	2
Canned, juice pack	1 cup	124	0.17/0	4	na	14 mcg (BC)	na	2	1	4	2
Canned, water pack	1 cup	71	0.1/0	4	na	0	na	3	1	2.4	2
Dried	10	459	1/t	13	na	na	na	0	t	12	0
Persimmons, medium	1 fruit	67	0/0	3.6	na	1.2 mg (BC) 1.5 mg (BCR)	na	7.2	0.4	7.2	0.6
						834 mcg (LU+Z)					
Pineapple:											
Fresh chunks	1 cup	76	0.67/0	2	104	19 mcg (BC)	na	17	1	24	0.3
Canned, heavy syrup, chunks, crushed, slices	1 cup	198	0.3/0	3	na	15 mcg (BC)	na	12	1	19	0.5
Canned, juice pack, chunks, crushed, slices	1 cup	150	0.2/0	2	na	60 mcg (BC)	na	12	1	24	0.3
Canned, light syrup, chunks, crushed, slices	1 cup	131	0.3/0	2	na	15 mcg (BC)	na	12	1	19	0.5
Canned, water pack, chunks, crushed, slices	1 cup	79	0.2/0	2	na	30 mcg (BC)	na	12	1	19	0.3

Food	Serving Size	Calories	Fat/Sat. Fat (gm)	Fiber (gm)	Flavonoids (mg)	Carotenoids (mcg or mg)	PE (mcg or mg)	Folate (mcg)	Selenium (mcg)	Vit. C (mg)	Vit. E (IUs)
Plaintains, raw	1 fruit	218	0.66/t	4	na	na	na	39	2.7	33	t
Plaintains, cooked	1 cup	176	0.28/t	3.5	na	na	na	40	2.2	17	t
Plums:											
Raw, medium	1 fruit	36	0.41/0	1	149	127 mcg (BC)	0	1	0.3	6.3	0.6
Canned, heavy syrup	1 cup	230	0.26/0	2.5	na	403 mcg (BC)	0	7	0.8	1	3
Canned, juice pack	1 cup	146	0.05/0	2.5	na	1.5 mg (BC)	0	8	0.8	7	2.5
Canned, light syrup	1 cup	159	0.3/0	2.5	na	393 mcg (BC)	na	7	0.8	1	3
Canned, water pack	1 cup	102	0/0	2.5	na	1.4 mg (BC)	na	6.5	0.7	7	2.5
Pomegranate, raw	1 fruit	105	0.5/0.1	0.9	na	0	na	9	0.9	9	1
Prunes:											
Dried, pitted, uncooked	5 prunes	100	0.22/0	3	na	502 mcg (BC)	5 mcg (D/G)	2	1	1.4	1
Stewed	1 cup	265	0.57/0	16	na	461 mcg (BC)	41 mcg (D/G)	0.2	2.5	7	0
Raisins	1 packet	42	0.06/t	0.6	na	na	26 mcg (D/G)	0	t	t	t
Raspberries:											
Raw	1 cup	60	0.68/0	8	na	15 mcg (AC) 96 mcg (BC)	171 mcg (L)	32	0.7	31	1
Frozen, sweetened	1 cup	258	0.4/0	11	na	90 mcg (BC)	na	65	1.5	41	1.5
Frozen, unsweetened	1 cup	123	1.4/0	17	na	185 mcg (BC)	na	62	1.5	44	1.5
Rhubarb, canned, light syrup	1 cup	220	0.2/0.1	3.5	na	120 mcg (BC)	na	15	2.4	9	0.6
Rhubarb, cooked, unsweetened	1 cup	50	0.5/0.1	4	na	108 mcg (BC)	na	8.5	3	13	0.75

154

Food	Serving Size	Calories	Fat/Sat.Fat (gm)	Fiber (gm)	Flavonoids (mg)	Carotenoids (mcg or mg)	PE (mcg or mg)	Folate (mcg)	Selenium (mcg)	Vit. C (mg)	Vit. E (IUs)
Strawberries:											
Raw	1 cup	50	0.61/0	4	220	8 mcg (AC) 30 mcg (BC)	8 mcg (D/G) 2.5 mg (L)	30	1.2	94	0.3
Frozen, sweetened	1 cup	222	0.33/0	5	na	38 mcg (BC)	na	24	1.8	103	0.75
Frozen, unsweetened	1 cup	77	0.2/0	5	na	53 mcg (BC)	na	37	1.5	91	1
Tangelo	1 fruit	45	0.1/0	2.3	na	120 mcg (BC)	na	29	0.5	51	0.3
Tangerine, medium	1	37	0.16/0	2	na	464 mcg (BC) 407 mcg (BCR) 204 mcg (LU+Z)	na	17	0.4	26	0.3
Tangerine (mandarin), canned, light syrup	1 cup	154	0.25/0	1.7	na	1.3 mg (BC)	na	12	1	50	1.4
Tangerine (mandarin), juice pack	1 cup	92	0.1/0	1.7	na	1.3 mg (BC)	na	12	1	85	2
Watermelon	1 wedge	92	1/0.1	1.4	80–183	844 mcg (BC) 14 mg (LYC)	na	6	0.3	27.5	0.6
GOOSE											
Roasted:											
Meat and skin	1 cup	427	31/10	0	0	0	0	2.8	30.5	0	4
Meat only	1 cup	340	18/6.5	0	0	0	0	17	36.5	0	na
Paté	1 tbsp.	60	5.7/1.8	0	0	0	0	8	5.7	0.26	na

Food	Serving Size	Calories	Fat/Sat. Fat (gm)	Fiber (gm)	Flavonoids (mg)	Carotenoids (mcg or mg)	PE (mcg or mg)	Folate (mcg)	Selenium (mcg)	Vit. C (mg)	Vit. E (IUs)
GRANOLA BARS											
Chewy	1 bar	126	5/2	1.3	na	na	na	7	4.6	0	na
Chewy w/ chocolate chips (Quaker Oats)	1 bar	127	5/4	1	na	2 mcg (BC)	na	23	4.5	0.3	0.3
Chewy w/ coconut	1 bar	195	7.6/5.5	1	na	2.4 mcg (BC)	na	35	7	0.4	0.45
Chocolate coated (Quaker Oats)	1 bar	130	6/3	1	na	2.4 mcg (BC)	na	8	2.5	0.7	0.75
Chocolate coated (Sweet Success)	1 bar	153	7/3	1	na	3 mcg (BC)	na	10	3	0.8	0.75
Chocolate coated, w/ nuts	1 bar	178	11/6	1	na	2.4 mcg (BC)	na	9	5.5	0.2	2
Coconut, chocolate coated	1 bar	198	13/9	2.4	na	5 mcg (BC)	na	3.5	6.4	0.2	1
Fruit and nut, lowfat (Nature Valley)	1 bar	106	2/0.2	1.5	na	284 mcg (BC)	na	45	4	0	0
Fruit, nuts, and oats, lowfat (Kellogg's)	1 bar	80	1/0.2	1	na	213 mcg (BC)	na	34	3	0	0
Non-chocolate coating (Quaker Oats)	1 bar	131	6/1	1	na	t (BC)	na	13	3	0.7	1.7
Nonfat (Health Valley) Fat-Free	1 bar	142	0.4/0.1	3	na	129 mcg (BC)	na	136	3.6	0.7	0.15
Nougat (Nature Valley Granola Cluster)	1 bar	138	4.5/2	1.4	na	2.4 mcg (BC)	na	11	2.5	0.2	2
Peanut butter (Nature Valley)	1 bar	90	3/0.5	1	na	na	na	na	na	0	na
Peanuts and wheat germ	1 bar	206	9/1	2	na	8 mcg (BC)	na	10	6.5	0	0.75

Food	Serving Size	Calories	Fat/Sat. Fat (gm)	Fiber (gm)	Flavonoids (mg)	Carotenoids (mcg or mg)	PE (mcg or mg)	Folate (mcg)	Selenium (mcg)	Vit. C (mg)	Vit. E (IUs)
Plain	1 bar	115	5/0.6	1.3	na	na	na	5.6	4	0.2	na
Rice-based (Kellogg's Rice Krispies bar)	1 bar	119	5/1.5	1	na	0	na	28	3.5	3.5	1
Trail mix, chewy (Quaker)	1 bar	130	5/0	t	na	na	na	na	na	na	na
Yogurt coated	1 bar	96	3/1	2.2	na	t (BC)	na	8	7.5	0.1	1
HOT DOGS											
Beef	1	185	17/7	0	0	0	0	2	8	0	0.15
Beef and pork	1	189	17/6	0	0	0	0	2	8	0	0.15
Beef, lowfat	1	136	11/5	0	0	0	0	2	8	0.5	0.15
Beef and pork, lowfat	1	92	6/2	0	0	0	0	2	9	0	0
Chicken	1	150	11/3	0	0	0	0	2	11	0	0.15
Chicken, beef, and pork	1	175	15/5	0	0	0	0	2	9	0	0.15
Light (Oscar Mayer)	1	110	8/3.5	0	0	0	0	na	na	0	na
Meat and poultry, fat-free (Ball Park or Oscar Mayer)	1	40	0/0	0	0	0	0	3	9	0	0
Meat and poultry, lowfat (Healthy Choice)	1	72	1.6/0.6	0	0	0	0	1.5	13	0.2	0.15
Meatless	1	140	7/1	3	0	0	na	55	5	0	2
Pork, light (Oscar Mayer)	1	111	8.5/3	0	0	0	0	na	na	0	0
Pork and turkey (Oscar Mayer)	1	145	13/4	0	0	0	0	na	na	0	na
3% fat (Hormel)	1	45	1/0	0	0	0	0	na	na	na	na

Food	Serving Size	Calories	Fat/Sat. Fat (gm)	Fiber (gm)	Flavonoids (mg)	Carotenoids (mcg or mg)	PE (mcg or mg)	Folate (mcg)	Selenium (mcg)	Vit. C (mg)	Vit. E (IUs)
Turkey	1	132	10/3.4	0	0	0	0	4	9	0	0.6
Turkey and chicken (Louis Rich)	1	85	6/2	0	0	0	0	na	na	0	na

ICE CREAM & FROZEN DESSERTS (REDUCED FAT)

Food	Serving Size	Calories	Fat/Sat. Fat (gm)	Fiber (gm)	Flavonoids (mg)	Carotenoids (mcg or mg)	PE (mcg or mg)	Folate (mcg)	Selenium (mcg)	Vit. C (mg)	Vit. E (IUs)
Dessert bar, frozen, fruit-flavored, low-calorie	1 bar	12	0.05/0	0	0	na	0	0	0.1	0	na
Dessert bar, frozen, nonfat, all flavors (Crystal Light)	1 bar	14	0/0	0	0	na	0	na	na	na	na
Dessert bar, frozen, nonfat, all flavors (Jell-O)	1 bar	35	0/0	0	0	na	0	na	na	na	na
Dessert bar, frozen, nonfat, double chocolate fudge (Light n' Lively)	1 bar	50	0/0	0	0	na	0	na	na	na	na
Dessert, frozen, nonfat (Sweet Nothings)	½ cup	100	0/0	0	0	na	0	na	na	na	na
Eskimo Pie, sugar-free	1 sandwich	184	5.4/2	0	0	1 mcg (BC)	0	18.5	3	0.1	1
Fruit bar, frozen, nonfat (Minute Maid)	1 bar	60	0/0	0	na	na	0	na	na	na	na
Fruit bar, frozen, nonfat, strawberry or raspberry (Dole)	1 bar	25	0/0	0	na	2.4 mcg (BC)	0	na	na	na	na

Food	Serving Size	Calories	Fat/Sat. Fat (gm)	Fiber (gm)	Flavonoids (mg)	Carotenoids (mcg or mg)	PE (mcg or mg)	Folate (mcg)	Selenium (mcg)	Vit. C (mg)	Vit. E (IUs)
Fudge pops, lowfat, low sugar (Fudgsicle)	1 bar	25	0.4/0.2	4.6	na	0	0	2.4	1	0.3	0
Ice cream, chocolate (Healthy Choice)	4 oz.	130	2/1	0	0	4 mcg (BC)	0	na	na	na	na
Ice cream, chocolate chip (Weight Watchers ONE-ders)	4 oz.	120	4/0	0	0	na	0	na	na	na	na
Ice cream, chocolate, lowfat (Haägen–Dazs)	½ cup	170	2.5/1.5	1	0	na	0	na	na	0	na
Ice cream, vanilla (Healthy Choice)	4 oz.	120	2/1	0	0	0	0	na	na	na	na
Ice cream, vanilla, light (Breyers)	½ cup	100	3/2	0	0	na	0	na	na	0	na
Ice cream, vanilla, lowfat (Haägen–Dazs)	½ cup	170	2.5/1.5	0	0	na	0	na	na	0	na
Ice cream, vanilla, no sugar (Edy's)	½ cup	80	3/1.5	na	0	na	0	na	na	0	na
Ice cream, vanilla, nonfat (Edy's)	½ cup	100	0/0	na	0	na	0	na	na	0	na
Ice milk bar (Weight Watchers)	1 bar	120	7/2	0	0	na	0	na	na	0	na
Ice milk, chocolate (Weight Watchers)	½ cup	110	3/2	0	0	8 mcg (BC)	0	na	na	na	na

159

Food	Serving Size	Calories	Fat/Sat. Fat (gm)	Fiber (gm)	Flavonoids (mg)	Carotenoids (mcg or mg)	PE (mcg or mg)	Folate (mcg)	Selenium (mcg)	Vit. C (mg)	Vit. E (IUs)
Ice milk, vanilla (Weight Watchers)	½ cup	100	3/1	0	0	8 mcg (BC)	0	na	na	na	na
Ice milk, vanilla, light	½ cup	92	3/2	0	0	na	0	4	2	0.5	0
Ice milk, vanilla, soft-serve, light	½ cup	111	2/1.4	0	0	21 mcg (BC)	0	5.3	3.6	0.8	0
Ice pop, frozen, w/ added vit. C	1 bar	42.5	0/0	0	0	0	0	0	0	6	na
Italian ice, cherry	1 cup	120	0/0	0	0	na	0	na	na	1	na
Nondairy dessert bar, frozen, chocolate (Rice Dream)	1 bar	270	16/0	0	0	na	na	na	na	na	na
Nondairy dessert bar, frozen, vanilla (Rice Dream)	1 bar	275	16/0	0	0	na	na	na	na	na	na
Nondairy dessert, carob or vanilla (Rice Dream)	½ cup	130	5/0	0	0	0.6 mcg (BC)	na	na	na	na	na
Praline caramel dessert (Healthy Choice)	½ cup	128.5	2/0.5	0	0	na	0	na	na	0	na
Praline toffee crunch parfait (Weight Watchers)	1 serving	190	3/0.2	2	0	na	0	na	na	0	na
Sherbet bar, frozen, all flavors, sugar-free (Fudgsicle)	1 bar	35	1/0	0	0	na	0	na	na	na	na
Sherbet bar, frozen, w/ cream, all flavors, sugar-free (Creamsicle)	1 bar	25	1/0	0	0	na	0	na	na	na	na

160

Food	Serving Size	Calories	Fat/Sat. Fat (gm)	Fiber (gm)	Flavonoids (mg)	Carotenoids (mcg or mg)	PE (mcg or mg)	Folate (mcg)	Selenium (mcg)	Vit. C (mg)	Vit. E (IUs)
Sherbet bar, frozen, all flavors, nonfat (Fudgsicle)	1 bar	70	0/0	0	0	na	0	na	na	na	na
Sorbet, orange, nonfat (Häagen Dazs)	½ cup	113	0/0	0	0	na	0	na	na	na	na
Sorbet, soft-serve, all flavors, nonfat (TCBY)	½ cup	100	0/0	0	0	na	0	na	na	0	na
LAMB											
Chop	1 medium chop	345	27/12	0	0	0	0	17.4	25	0	0.15
Leg, roasted	3 oz.	199	12/6	0	0	0	0	0.9	3.5	0	0.2
Rib, roasted	3 oz.	290	23/10	0	0	0	0	13.6	19	0	0.14
Shoulder, roasted	3 oz.	241	13.5/5	0	0	0	0	18	31.5	0	0.25
Sweetbreads	3 oz.	148	3.6/1.3	0	0	0	0	0.9	83	63	1
MILK & MILK BEVERAGES											
Buttermilk, cultured	1 cup	90	1/0	0	0	0	0	na	na	na	na
Chocolate milk:											
1% Lowfat	1 cup	158	2.5/1.5	1.25	0	0	0	12	4.75	2	0.1
2% Reduced fat	1 cup	190	5/0	0	0	0	0	12	4.75	na	0.2
Whole	1 cup	210	8/0	0	0	0	0	12	4.75	na	0.3
Milk:											
Instant nonfat (dried), prepared	1 cup	80	0/0	0	0	0	0	na	na	na	na

161

Food	Serving Size	Calories	Fat/Sat. Fat (gm)	Fiber (gm)	Flavonoids (mg)	Carotenoids (mcg or mg)	PE (mcg or mg)	Folate (mcg)	Selenium (mcg)	Vit. C (mg)	Vit. E (IUs)
Lowfat (1%)	1 cup	100–104	2/0	0	0	0	0	13	5.6	na	0.15
Nonfat	1 cup	90	0/0	0	0	0	0	13	5.4	na	0.15
Reduced fat (2%)	1 cup	121	4.6/1.3	0	0	0	0	12.5	5.4	2.3	0.25
Whole	1 cup	150	8/5	0	0	0	0	12	5	2.3	0.4
Milk, evaporated:											
Lowfat (Carnation)	½ cup	110	3/2	0	0	0	0	10	na	0.8	na
Regular (Carnation)	½ cup	170	10/0	0	0	0	0	na	na	na	na
Milk, goat's	1 cup	168	10/3	0	0	0	0	1.5	3.4	3	0.3
Sweetened, condensed	1 fl. oz.	123	3.3/2	0	0	0	0	4	5.6	1	0.1
Eggnog, nonalcoholic	1 cup	350	17/0	0	0	0	0	na	na	na	na
Hot cocoa, prepared with water (Swiss Miss)	1 packet	110	3/1.3	0	0	0	0	na	na	na	na
Hot cocoa, prepared with water, sugar-free (Swiss Miss)	1 packet	48	0.46/0.27	0.36	0	0	0	2.2	2.7	0	0.09
Instant Breakfast, made with 2% milk (Carnation)	9 oz.	250	5/0	na	0	0	0	92	na	30	7.5
Instant Breakfast, made with 2% milk, sugar-free (Carnation)	9 oz.	190	5/0	na	0	0	0	92	na	30	7.5
Malted milk, fortified, prepared with whole milk	1 cup	225	9/5.5	0.27	0	0	0	32	6.3	34	na

Food	Serving Size	Calories	Fat/Sat. Fat (gm)	Fiber (gm)	Flavonoids (mg)	Carotenoids (mcg or mg)	PE (mcg or mg)	Folate (mcg)	Selenium (mcg)	Vit. C (mg)	Vit. E (IUs)
Milkshake, chocolate	11 oz.	356	8/5	0.9	0	0	0	15	5.7	0	0.5
Milkshake, vanilla	11 oz.	350	9.5/6	0	0	0	0	21	7	0	0.5
NUTS, SEEDS, & PRODUCTS											
Almonds:											
Butter	1 tbsp.	101	9.5/0.9	0.6	na	0	na	10.5	0.12	0.11	**5**
Dry roasted, salted	22 nuts (1 oz.)	169	15/1	3.4	na	0	33.5 mg	9.4	2.2	0	**11**
Oil roasted, salted	22 nuts (1 oz.)	172	16/1.2	3	na	0	37 mg	7.7	2.2	0	**11**
Slivered	1 cup	624	55/4	**13**	na	0	130 mg	31	8.5	0	**42**
Brazil nuts	6–8 nuts	186	19/5	1.5	na	0	na	1.1	839	0.2	3
Cashews:											
Butter	1 tbsp.	94	8/1.6	0.32	na	0	na	11	2	0	0.4
Dry roasted, salted	18 nuts (1 oz.)	163	13/2.6	0.85	na	0	45 mg	19.6	3.3	0	0.24
Oil roasted, salted	18 nuts (1 oz.)	164	14/3	1	na	0	45 mg	19	3.2	0	0.7
Chestnuts	10 nuts	206	2/0.3	4.3	na	10 mcg (BC)	na	59	1	22	1.5
Coconut:											
Raw	1 piece, 2 x 2 x ½"	159	15/13	4	na	0	21 mg	12	4.5	1.5	0.5
Shredded, sweetened	1 oz.	135	9/8	1.2	na	0	na	2.2	4.6	0	0.3
Shredded, unsweetened	1 oz.	187	18/16	4.6	na	0	na	2.5	5	0.4	0.6

Food	Serving Size	Calories	Fat/Sat. Fat (gm)	Fiber (gm)	Flavonoids (mg)	Carotenoids (mcg or mg)	PE (mcg or mg)	Folate (mcg)	Selenium (mcg)	Vit. C (mg)	Vit. E (IUs)
Flaxseed	1 tbsp.	59	4/0.4	3.4	na	0	52 mg (L)	33	0.66	0.16	1
Hazelnuts	10 nuts	88	8.5/0.6	1.4	na	6.6 mcg (BC)	13.4 mg	16	0.6	0.9	3
Macadamia nuts:											
Dry roasted, salted	10–12 nuts (1 oz.)	203	22/4	2.3	na	1.8 mcg (BC)	32 mg	3	1	0.2	0.24
Mixed nuts:											
Dry roasted, salted	1 oz.	168	15/2	2.5	na	1.8 mcg (BC)	na	14	2	0.11	2.5
Oil roasted, salted	1 oz.	174	16/2.6	1.6	na	3.6 mcg (BC)	na	16	118	0.14	2.5
Peanuts:											
Boiled	About 33 nuts (1 oz.)	89	6/0.9	2.5	na	0	na	21	1.2	0	1.4
Dry roasted, salted	1 oz.	166	14/2	2.3	na	0	42 mcg (L)	41	2	0	3
Honey roasted	1 oz.	153	12/2	2.3	na	0	na	31	2	0	3
Oil roasted	1 oz.	163	14/2	2.6	na	0	42 mcg (L)	35	2	0	3
Spanish, oil roasted	1 oz.	164	14/2	2.5	na	0	na	36	2	0	na
Peanut butter:											
Chunky	2 tbsp.	188.5	16/3	2	na	0	33 mg	30	2.4	0	na
Reduced fat	2 tbsp.	187	12/2.6	2	na	0	na	22	2.6	0	3.6
Smooth	2 tbsp.	190	16/3	1.8	na	0	33 mg	24	2.4	0	5
Pecans:											
Dried	20 halves (1 oz.)	196	20/2	3	na	22 mcg (BC)	29 mg	6	1.7	0.3	1.5

Food	Serving Size	Calories	Fat/Sat. Fat (gm)	Fiber (gm)	Flavonoids (mg)	Carotenoids (mcg or mg)	PE (mcg or mg)	Folate (mcg)	Selenium (mcg)	Vit. C (mg)	Vit. E (IUs)
Dry roasted, salted	20 halves (1 oz.)	201	21/1.8	2.7	na	22 mcg (BC)	24 mg	4.5	1.13	0.3	1.5
Oil roasted, salted	15 halves (1 oz.)	203	21/2	2.7	na	na	31 mg	4.3	1.7	0.3	2
Pine nuts	10 nuts	6	0.6/0.09	0.1	na	0.6 mcg (BC)	na	0.6	na	0.02	na
Pistachios, dry roasted	47 nuts (1 oz.)	161	13/1.6	3	na	40 mcg (BC)	61 mg	14	2.3	0.7	2
Pumpkin seeds, dried	1 oz.	146	12/2	1	na	64 mcg (BC)	na	16	1.6	0.5	0.5
Sesame seeds, dry	1 tbsp.	47	4.4/0.6	1	na	t	na	7.7	0.14	0	0.3
Sunflower seeds, hulled:											
Dry roasted	1 oz.	93	8/0.8	1.4	na	0	85 mcg (L)	38	12.7	0.2	12
Oil roasted	1 oz.	105	10/1	1.2	na	5.4 mcg (BC)	85 mcg (L)	40	13	0.2	11
Tahini (sesame butter)	1 tbsp.	85.5	7/1	1.4	na	6.6 mcg (BC)	na	14.7	na	0	na
Trail Mix:											
Regular	1 cup	693	44/8	9	na	11 mcg (BC)	na	130	23.6	2	23
With chocolate chips	1 cup	707	47/9	na	na	na	na	95	na	2	na
Tropical	1 cup	570	24/12	na	na	na	112 mg	59	na	11	na
Walnuts:											
Black	14 halves (1 oz.)	172	16/1	1.4	na	20 mcg (BC)	23 mcg (L)	18.5	5	1	1
English	14 halves (1 oz.)	185	18.5/1.7	2	na	20 mcg (BC)	20 mg	28	1.3	0.4	1

PANCAKES, WAFFLES, & FRENCH TOAST

Food	Serving Size	Calories	Fat/Sat Fat (gm)	Fiber (gm)	Flavonoids (mg)	Carotenoids (mcg or mg)	PE (mcg or mg)	Folate (mcg)	Selenium (mcg)	Vit. C (mg)	Vit. E (IIUs)
French toast, from recipe, w/ 2% milk	1 slice	149	7/1.7	na	0	na	na	28	**13**	0.2	na
French toast, ready-to-heat	1 piece	126	3.6/0.9	0.65	0	1.2 mcg	na	31	10	0.18	0.6
Pancakes:											
Blueberry	1 pancake, 6" dia.	105	3.5/1	1	na	10 mcg	na	17	5	1.5	0.75
Buckwheat	1 pancake, 6" dia.	98	3.5/1	1.4	0	3.6 mcg	na	9.6	5	0.3	0.6
Buttermilk, Eggo (Kellogg's)	1 serving	233	6.7/1.4	1	0	na	na	52	na	1.4	0
Buttermilk, from recipe	1 pancake, 6" dia.	175	7/1.4	na	0	na	na	29	12	0.3	na
Cornmeal	1 pancake, 6" dia.	112	3.3/0.8	1	0	55 mcg	na	27	5	0.1	0.6
Plain	1 pancake, 6" dia.	126	1.8/0.4	1	0	9 mcg	na	25	8.6	0.2	0.6
Plain, ready-to-head, from frozen	1 pancake, 6" dia.	167	2.4/0.5	1.3	0	na	na	36.5	8.6	0.2	0.44
Reduced calorie (Aunt Jemima Lite)	1 pancake, 6" dia.	117	2.2/0.6	4.4	0	6.6 mcg	na	25	8.4	0.5	0.75
Rye	1 pancake, 6" dia.	165	6/1.3	2	0	1.2 mcg	na	16.5	11	0.2	1.2

166

Food	Serving Size	Calories	Fat/Sat. Fat (gm)	Fiber (gm)	Flavonoids (mg)	Carotenoids (mcg or mg)	PE (mcg or mg)	Folate (mcg)	Selenium (mcg)	Vit. C (mg)	Vit. E (IUs)
Sourdough	1 pancake, 6" dia.	121	3.6/0.7	0.8	0	0	na	38	9.4	0	1.4
Whole wheat	1 pancake, 6" dia.	127	5.6/1.2	2	0	4 mcg	na	9	15	0.3	1.7
Waffles:											
Banana bread, Nutri-Grain (Kellogg's)	1 serving	212	7.4/1.3	2	na	na	na	40	na	1	0
Blueberry, Eggo (Kellogg's)	1 serving	73	1/0.14	1	na	0	na	18	na	0	na
Frozen (Aunt Jemima)	1 serving	197	6/1.6	na	na	0	na	na	na	na	na
Golden Oat, Eggo (Kellogg's)	1 serving	137	2.2/0.4	2.5	na	0	na	29	na	0.6	na
Homestyle, lowfat, Eggo (Kellogg's)	1 serving	165	2.5/0.6	0.7	0	0	na	54	na	0	na
Nutri-Grain, Eggo (Kellogg's)	1 serving	142	2.2/0.3	2.6	0	0	na	36	na	0	na
Plain, fat-free	1 serving	74	0.1/0	0.4	0	0	na	14	7	0	0
Plain, lowfat	1 serving	87	0.7/0.1	0.4	0	0	na	14.5	6	0.1	0.15
Plain, from recipe	1 waffle, 7" dia.	218	11/2	na	0	0	na	34.5	35	0.3	na
Plain, ready-to-heat, from frozen	1 waffle, 4" sq.	88	3/0.5	0.8	0	0	na	18.5	6.5	0	0.7
Toaster	1 waffle, 4" sq.	87	2.7/0.5	0.8	0	0	na	15	5	0	0.4

167

Food	Serving Size	Calories	Fat/Sat. Fat (gm)	Fiber (gm)	Flavonoids (mg)	Carotenoids (mcg or mg)	PE (mcg or mg)	Folate (mcg)	Selenium (mcg)	Vit. C (mg)	Vit. E (IUs)
PASTA & NOODLES (COOKED)											
Chinese noodles, chow mein	1 cup	237	14/2	2	0	0	na	40.5	19.4	0	0.1
Corn-based pasta	1 cup	176	1/0.14	7	0	42 mcg	na	8	4	0	0.7
Egg noodles, enriched	1 cup	213	2.4/0.5	2	0	0	na	102	35	0	0.12
Egg noodles, spinach, enriched	1 cup	211	2.5/0.6	3.7	na	na	na	102	35	0	0.12
Japanese noodles, soba	1 cup	113	0.1/0.02	na	na	na	na	8	na	0	na
Japanese noodles, somen	1 cup	231	0.3/0.04	na	na	na	na	3.5	na	0	na
Macaroni, elbow	1 cup	197	1/0.3	2	0	0	na	98	30	0	0.06
Macaroni, spinach	1 cup	191	0.8/0.1	5.4	na	44 mcg	na	17	33	0	0
Macaroni, vegetable	1 cup	171	0.15/0.02	6	na	na	na	87	26.5	0	0.08
Macaroni, elbows, whole wheat	1 cup	174	0.75/0.14	4	0	0	na	7	36	0	0.2
Pasta, fresh	1 cup	262	2/0.3	na	0	0	na	128	na	0	na
Pasta, fresh, spinach	1 cup	260	2/0.4	na	na	na	na	128	na	0	na
Pasta, linguini	1 cup	197	0.9/0.1	2.4	0	0	na	98	30	0	0.15
Rice noodles	1 cup	192	0.35/0.04	2	0	0	na	5	8	0	na
Spaghetti, enriched	1 cup	230	0.3/0.04	3	0	0	na	115	35	0	na
Spaghetti, enriched, spinach	1 cup	182	0.9/0.12	na	0	na	na	17	31	0	na
Spaghetti, enriched, whole wheat	1 cup	174	0.75/0.14	6	0	0	na	7	36	0	0.1

Food	Serving Size	Calories	Fat/Sat. Fat (gm)	Fiber (gm)	Flavonoids (mg)	Carotenoids (mcg or mg)	PE (mcg or mg)	Folate (mcg)	Selenium (mcg)	Vit. C (mg)	Vit. E (IUs)
PORK/HAM											
Boneless	3 oz.	149	7.6/1.7	0	0	0	0	3	20	23	5.3
Canned, extra lean	3 oz.	142	7/2.4	0	0	0	0	4	23	0	0.33
Patty, grilled	1 patty	203	18/6.7	0	0	0	0	1.8	12.5	0	0.23
Roasted, lean portion	3 oz.	206	14/5	0	0	0	0	2.5	19	0	0.33
PORK/PORK											
Center rib, broiled	3 oz.	184	8.5/3	0	0	0	0	7.7	40	0.25	na
Chop, lean, breaded or floured, broiled or baked	1 med. (5.5 oz.)	207	8.4/3	0.2	0	94 mcg	0	10.5	41	0.8	0.45
Chop, lean, broiled or baked	1 med. (5.5 oz.)	176	8/3	0	0	0	0	5	40.5	0.6	0.3
Cutlet, lean, broiled or baked	3 oz.	181	9/3	0	0	0	0	5	36	0.6	0.3
Ground patty	1 patty	297	21/8	0	0	0	0	6	35	0.7	0.45
Roast, lean, loin	3 oz.	178	8/3	0	0	0	0	4	30	0.5	0.3
Roast, lean, shoulder	3 oz.	196	11.5/4	0	0	0	0	4	32	0.5	0.3
Spareribs, lean	1 med. cut	161	7/3	0	0	0	0	1.6	34	0.2	0.3
Tenderloin, baked	3 oz.	147	5/2	0	0	0	0	5	40	0.3	0.3
PORK/PORK PRODUCTS											
Bacon, Canadian style	2 slices	86	4/1.3	0	0	0	0	2	11.5	0	0.18
Bacon	3 slices	109	9.4/3	0	0	0	0	1	5	0	0.15
Breakfast strips	3 slices	156	12.5/4	0	0	0	0	1	8.4	0	0.15

169

Food	Serving Size	Calories	Fat/Sat. Fat (gm)	Fiber (gm)	Flavonoids (mg)	Carotenoids (mcg or mg)	PE (mcg or mg)	Folate (mcg)	Selenium (mcg)	Vit. C (mg)	Vit. E (IUs)
PORK/VARIETY MEATS											
Pork feet, pickled	1 oz.	75	5/2	0	0	0	0	0.6	35	0	na
Tongue, braised	3 oz.	271	18.6/6.5	0	0	0	0	4	15.5	1.7	na
PUDDING											
Banana:											
Instant, prep. w/ 2% milk	½ cup	153	2.5/1.5	0	na	na	na	6	2.7	1.2	na
Instant, sugar-free, prep. w/ 2% milk (Jell-O)	½ cup	80	2/0	0	na	9 mcg (BC)	na	na	na	na	na
Ready to eat	½ cup	158	6/2	0	na	13 mcg (BC)	na	na	na	0	na
Regular, prep. w/ 2% milk	½ cup	143	2.4/1.5	0	na	na	na	6	2.7	1	na
Bread pudding, w/ raisins	1 cup	310	10/3.4	2	na	49 mcg (BC)	na	37	19	1.3	1.7
Butterscotch:											
Instant, sugar-free, prep. w/ 2% milk (Jell-O)	½ cup	90	2/0	0	na	9 mcg (BC)	na	na	na	na	na
Low-calorie, prep. w/ skim milk (D-Zerta)	½ cup	70	0/0	0	na	na	na	na	na	na	na
Ready to eat (Musselman's)	½ cup	170	7/0	0	na	13 mcg (BC)	na	na	na	na	na
Ready to eat (Ultra Slim•Fast)	½ cup	100	1/0	2	na	0	na	na	na	na	na
Chocolate:											
Instant, prep. w/ 2% milk	½ cup	150	3/1.6	0.6	na	na	na	6	2.5	1.3	na

170

Food	Serving Size	Calories	Fat/Sat. Fat (gm)	Fiber (gm)	Flavonoids (mg)	Carotenoids (mcg or mg)	PE (mcg or mg)	Folate (mcg)	Selenium (mcg)	Vit. C (mg)	Vit. E (IUs)
Instant, sugar-free, prep. w/ 2% milk (Jell-O)	½ cup	90	3/0	0	na	10 mcg (BC)	na	na	na	na	na
Lower fat (D-Zerta)	1 serving	20	0/0	0.5	na	0	na	0.3	na	0	na
Ready to eat	½ cup	133	4/1	1	na	13 mcg (BC)	na	3	1.5	2	0.2
Ready to eat, fat-free (Jell-O)	½ cup	90	0.4/0.3	0.8	na	0	na	na	na	0.3	na
Regular, prep. w/ 2% milk	½ cup	150	3/2	0.5	na	na	na	6	2.6	1	na
Coconut cream:											
Instant, prep. w/ 2% milk	½ cup	157	3.4/2	0.15	na	na	na	6	3	1.2	na
Regular, prep. w/ 2% milk	½ cup	146	3.5/2.5	0.3	na	na	na	6	3	1	0.15
Custard:											
Mix, prep. w/ 2% milk	½ cup	149	4/2	0	na	na	na	11	na	1	na
Mix, prep. w/ whole milk (Royal)	½ cup	150	5/0	0	na	12 mcg (BC)	na	na	na	na	na
Flan:											
Mix, prep. w/ 2% milk	½ cup	136	2.4/1.5	0.13	na	na	na	5	7	1	na
Mix, prep. w/ whole milk	½ cup	150	4/2.5	0.13	na	6 mcg (BC)	na	5	6.5	1	na
Key Lime: prep. w/ whole milk (Royal)	½ cup	160	3/0	0	na	na	na	na	na	na	na
Lemon:											
Instant, prep. w/ 2% milk	½ cup	154	2.5/1.5	0	na	na	na	6	3	1	na
Ready to eat	½ cup	138	3/1	0	na	13 mcg (BC)	na	na	na	0	na

Food	Serving Size	Calories	Fat/Sat. Fat (gm)	Fiber (gm)	Flavonoids (mg)	Carotenoids (mcg or mg)	PE (mcg or mg)	Folate (mcg)	Selenium (mcg)	Vit. C (mg)	Vit. E (IUs)
Regular, prep. w/ whole milk (Royal)	½ cup	160	3/0	0	na	na	na	na	na	na	na
Medical Puddings:											
Boost Pudding	5 oz.	240	9/1.5	0	na	na	na	60	na	9	4.5
Ensure Pudding	4 oz.	170	5/1	na	na	na	na	60	8	9	3
Pistachio:											
Instant, prep. w/ whole milk (Jell-O)	½ cup	170	5/0	0	na	na	na	na	na	na	na
Instant, sugar-free, prep. w/ 2% milk (Jell-O)	½ cup	90	3/0	0	na	9 mcg (BC)	na	na	na	na	na
Rice:											
Ready to eat (Musselman's)	½ cup	120	3/0	0	na	11 mcg (BC)	na	na	na	na	na
Regular, prep. w/ 2% milk	½ cup	161	2.3/1.5	0.15	na	11 mcg (BC)	na	6	3	1	na
Tapioca:											
Light, ready to eat (Swiss Miss)	½ cup	100	2/0	0	na	na	na	na	na	na	na
Nonfat, ready to eat (Snack Pack)	½ cup	94	0.4/0	0	na	0	na	na	na	0	na
Ready to eat, regular (Lucky Leaf)	½ cup	140	6/0	0	na	9 mcg (BC)	na	na	na	na	na

172

Food	Serving Size	Calories	Fat/Sat. Fat (gm)	Fiber (gm)	Flavonoids (mg)	Carotenoids (mcg or mg)	PE (mcg or mg)	Folate (mcg)	Selenium (mcg)	Vit. C (mg)	Vit. E (IUs)
Regular, prep. w/ 2% milk	½ cup	147	2.4/1.5	0	na	na	na	6	3	1	na
Vanilla:											
Instant, sugar-free, prep. w/ 2% milk (Jell-O)	½ cup	90	2/0	0	na	na	na	na	na	na	na
Low-calorie, prep. w/ nonfat milk (D-Zerta)	½ cup	70	0/0	0	na	9 mcg (BC)	na	na	na	na	na
Ready to eat	½ cup	180	7/0	0	na	na	na	na	na	na	na
Ready to eat, fat-free (Jell-O)	½ cup	92	0.2/0.2	0.1	na	13 mcg (BC)	na	na	na	0.3	na
Ready to eat, light (Ultra Slim•Fast)	½ cup	100	1/0	2	na	0	na	na	na	na	na
Regular, prep. w/ 2% milk	½ cup	141	2.4/1.5	0	na	0	na	6	3	1	na
SALADS*											
7-layer salad	1 cup	197	14/4	2	na	169 mcg (BC)	na	39	5	9	2
Apple salad	1 cup	192	13/2	3	na	49 mcg (BC)	na	16	1	7	2
Bean salad	1 cup	70	4/0.6	3	na	48 mcg (BC)	na	28	0.7	2	1.4
Broccoli salad w/ cauliflower	1 cup	428	37/9	3	na	293 mcg (BC)	na	59	5	43	8

*All salads are prepared with fat-based dressings, unless otherwise specified.

Food	Serving Size	Calories	Fat/Sat. Fat (gm)	Fiber (gm)	Flavonoids (mg)	Carotenoids (mcg or mg)	PE (mcg or mg)	Folate (mcg)	Selenium (mcg)	Vit. C (mg)	Vit. E (IUs)
Caesar salad	1 cup	168	14/3	1.4	na	1 mg (BC)	na	105	8	19	3
Carrot salad w/ raisins	1 cup	419	30/5	4	na	16 mg (BC)	na	18	2	13	7.5
Chef salad w/o dressing	1 cup	73	4/2	0.6	na	519 mcg (BC)	na	28	9	3	0.45
Chicken salad	5 oz.	290	22/4	0.5	na	22 mcg (BC)	na	24	21	3	4
Cobb salad	1 cup	180	15/4	2	na	595 mcg (BC)	na	65	8	12	3
Coleslaw	1 cup	271	24/4	4	na	2.6 mg (BC)	na	60	2	42	6
Crab salad	5 oz.	211	10/2	0.5	na	24 mcg (BC)	na	60	41	5	3
Crab salad w/ imitation crab	5 oz.	224	9/1	0.6	na	24 mcg (BC)	na	11	26	2	2
Cranberry salad, jellied	1 cup	348	12/1	5	na	55 mcg (BC)	na	25	3	17	1
Egg salad	½ cup	354	34/6	0	na	0	na	37	25	0	7
Fruit salad w/ citrus	1 cup	152	8/2	3	na	80 mcg (BC)	na	30	2	57	2
Fruit salad w/o citrus	1 cup	184	8/2	4	na	56 mcg (BC)	na	19	2	16	2
Greek salad	1 cup	106	7/4	1	na	404 mcg (BC)	na	45	12	6	1.4
Ham salad	5 oz.	298	23/4	0.6	na	26 mcg (BC)	na	15	21	2	5
Macaroni salad	1 cup	271	9/1	2	na	35 mcg (BC)	na	84	23	2	1.7
Mixed salad greens, raw, w/o dressing	1 cup	9	0.1/0	1	na	898 mcg (BC)	na	64	0.2	9	0.6
Pasta salad w/ vegetables	1 cup	287	16/2	2	na	2.4 mg (BC)	na	75	20	12	5
Pea salad	1 cup	501	43/7	7	na	541 mcg (BC)	na	83	10	44	10
Pear salad	½ pear, lettuce	117	6/0.8	2	na	22 mcg (BC)	na	11	1	4	1.7

Food	Serving Size	Calories	Fat/Sat. Fat (gm)	Fiber (gm)	Flavonoids (mg)	Carotenoids (mcg or mg)	PE (mcg or mg)	Folate (mcg)	Selenium (mcg)	Vit. C (mg)	Vit. E (IUs)
Pineapple salad	1 cup diced fruit, lettuce	141	6/0.8	2	na	30 mcg (BC)	na	21	1	25	1
Potato salad	1 cup	139	8/1	2	na	34 mcg (BC)	na	11	0.8	12	2
Potato salad, German	1 cup	155	3/1	3	na	35 mcg (BC)	na	19	2	19	0.15
Shrimp salad	5 oz.	212	13/2	0.6	na	27 mcg (BC)	na	12	34	4	4
Spinach salad w/o dressing	1 cup	108	5/1	2	na	870 mcg (BC)	na	67	13	7	1.4
Taco salad w/ beef, fried flour tortilla	1 salad	435	29/11	4	na	398 mcg (BC)	na	85	20	13	3.5
Tomato and cucumber salad	1 cup	185	16/2	na	na	219 mcg (BC)	na	15	0.3	12	5
Tuna salad	5 oz.	222	8/1	0.7	na	31 mcg (BC)	na	11	68	2	2
SALAD DRESSINGS/FAT-FREE											
1,000 Island	1 tbsp.	18	0.3/0	0	0	2.4 mcg (BC)	4 mg	0.5	0.3	0.1	0.15
Blue cheese	1 tbsp.	19	0.1/0	0.6	0	6 mcg (BC)	na	0.5	0.3	0	0.15
Creamy, various brands	1 tbsp.	12	0.6/0.4	0	0	1 mcg (BC)	na	0.6	0.2	0.1	0
French	1 tbsp.	21	0.5/0.1	0	0	125 mcg (BC)	na	0	0.3	0	0.2
Italian	1 tbsp.	6	0.3/0	0	0	2 mcg (BC)	na	2	0.2	0.1	0.15
Mayo-type, various brands	1 tbsp.	12	0.4/0.1	0.6	0	0	na	0	0.3	0	0.45
Ranch	1 tbsp.	18	0.4/0.1	0	0	0	na	0.5	0.3	0	0.1
Russian	1 tbsp.	23	0.65/0.09	0.05	0	0	1.6 mg	0.6	0.3	1	0.19
Sweet and sour	1 tbsp.	3	0/0	0	0	1 mcg (BC)	na	0.5	0.2	1.3	0
Vinaigrette	1 tbsp.	8	0/0	0	0	0	na	0	0	0	0

Food	Serving Size	Calories	Fat/Sat. Fat (gm)	Fiber (gm)	Flavonoids (mg)	Carotenoids (mcg or mg)	PE (mcg or mg)	Folate (mcg)	Selenium (mcg)	Vit. C (mg)	Vit. E (IUs)
SALAD DRESSING/REDUCED CALORIE											
1,000 Island	1 tbsp.	24	1.6/0.2	0.2	0	0	4 mg	0.9	0.2	0	0.3
Bacon & tomato	1 tbsp.	32.4	3.4/0.5	0	0	26.4 mcg (BC)	na	0	0.3	1.4	0.9
Blue cheese	1 tbsp.	15	1.1/0.4	0	0	0	na	0.5	0.2	0	0.15
Buttermilk	1 tbsp.	31	3/0.6	0	0	1 mcg (BC)	1 mg	0.2	0	0.1	0.96
Caesar	1 tbsp.	16.5	0.7/0.1	0	0	2 mcg (BC)	na	0.3	0.2	0	0.15
Coleslaw	1 tbsp.	34	3.4/0.5	0.1	0	0	na	0.5	0.3	0	1
Creamy, cholesterol-free (Hidden Valley Take Heart brands)	1 tbsp.	21	1/0.2	0	0	0	na	0.5	0.2	0	0.1
Creamy cucumber	1 tbsp.	24	2/0.3	0	0	6.6 mcg (BC)	na	2	0.2	0.1	0.45
Dijon vinaigrette, light (Wish-Bone)	1 tbsp.	16	1.5/0.2	0	0	0	na	0	0.2	0	0.3
French	1 tbsp.	32	2/0.3	0	0	127 mcg (BC)	na	0	0.3	0	0.3
Imitation mayonnaise	1 tbsp.	38	3/0.4	0	0	0	0.9 mg	0.9	0.2	0	0.9
Italian	1 tbsp.	28	3/0.4	0	0	2 mcg (BC)	4 mg	2	0.2	0.1	0.1
Ranch	1 tbsp.	26	2/0.2	0.2	0	0	1.6 mg	2	0	0.25	0
Russian	1 tbsp.	23	0.6/0.1	0	0	0	na	0.6	0.3	1	0.15
SALAD DRESSINGS/REGULAR											
1,000 Island	1 tbsp.	59	5.6/0.9	0	0	0	15 mg	1	0.3	0	0.3
Bacon (hot)	1 tbsp.	101	11/1.7	0	0	0	na	0.1	0.7	0	2.7
Bacon & tomato	1 tbsp.	49	5/0.8	0	0	24.6 mcg	na	0	0.2	1.3	0.9

Food	Serving Size	Calories	Fat/Sat. Fat (gm)	Fiber (gm)	Flavonoids (mg)	Carotenoids (mcg or mg)	PE (mcg or mg)	Folate (mcg)	Selenium (mcg)	Vit. C (mg)	Vit. E (IUs)
Blue cheese	1 tbsp.	77	8/1.5	0	0	0	20 mg	1.2	0.2	0.3	2
Boiled, cooked-type	1 tbsp.	25	1.5/0.5	0	0	118 mcg (BC)	na	1.4	0.3	0.1	0.45
Caesar	1 tbsp.	78	8.5/1.3	0	0	2 mcg (BC)	na	0.3	0.2	0	0.96
Celery seed	1 tbsp.	98	9.6/1.2	0.2	0	58 mcg (BC)	na	1.5	0.1	0.8	2.85
Coleslaw	1 tbsp.	121	10/1.5	0	0	3.6 mcg (BC)	na	2	0	0	3
Creamy Italian or cucumber	1 tbsp.	74	8/1	0	0	2 mcg (BC)	na	0.2	0.5	0	2.3
Feta cheese (Marzetti)	1 tbsp.	80	8.6/1.7	0	0	1 mcg (BC)	na	1.4	0.7	0.1	1.5
French	1 tbsp.	67	6.4/1.5	0	0	122 mcg (BC)	16 mg	0.7	0.2	0	2
Green goddess	1 tbsp.	78	7.6/1	0	0	9 mcg (BC)	na	0.6	0.2	0	1.8
Honey mustard	1 tbsp.	51	3/0.3	0	0.1	0	na	0.5	1	0.1	0.9
Italian	1 tbsp.	69	7/1	0	0	0	18 mg	0.7	0.2	0	2.3
Mayo-type (Miracle Whip)	1 tbsp.	57	5/0.7	0	0	0	48 mg	0.9	0.2	0	0.9
Mayo-type, cholesterol-free (Miracle Whip)	1 tbsp.	103	12/1.6	0	0	0	na	0	0.2	0	2.7
Peppercorn	1 tbsp.	76	8/1.4	0	0	2 mcg (BC)	na	3.6	0.2	0.1	0.6
Poppy seed	1 tbsp.	65	6/0.9	0	0	0	na	0.2	0	0	1.65
Ranch	1 tbsp.	74	8/1	0.45	0	0	na	0	0	0.25	0
Russian	1 tbsp.	76	8/1	0	0	0	19 mg	1.6	0.2	0.9	2.4
Sesame seed	1 tbsp.	78	8/1	0.1	0	3.6 mcg (BC)	17 mg	0.1	0.2	0	0.6
Vinaigrette	1 tbsp.	69	7/1	0	0	0	na	0.7	0.2	0	2.3
Yogurt	1 tbsp.	11	0.6/0.3	0	0	2.4 mcg (BC)	na	1	0.3	0.4	0
Zesty Italian (Kraft)	1 tbsp.	54	6.5/0.5	0.08	0	0	na	0	0	0.08	0

Food	Serving Size	Calories	Fat/Sat. Fat (gm)	Fiber (gm)	Flavonoids (mg)	Carotenoids (mcg or mg)	PE (mcg or mg)	Folate (mcg)	Selenium (mcg)	Vit. C (mg)	Vit. E (IUs)
SANDWICH MEATS, LEAN											
Beef lunch meat, lean	1 oz.	40	2/0	0	0	0	0	na	na	na	na
Bologna, 15% chicken	1 oz.	90	8/0	0	0	0	0	na	na	na	na
Bologna, chicken (Health Valley)	1 slice	85	8/0	0	0	0	0	na	na	na	na
Bologna, fat-free (Oscar Mayer)	1 slice	22	0.2/t	0	0	0	0	na	na	0	na
Bologna, light (Oscar Mayer)	1 slice	60	4/1.5	0	0	0	0	na	na	0	na
Bologna, lowfat (Healthy Choice)	1 slice	30	1/0.5	0	0	0	0	na	na	2.4	na
Bologna, turkey	1 slice	56	4/1.5	0	0	0	0	2	3.5	0	0.2
Chicken breast, baked (Louis Rich)	1 slice	21.5	0.1/0.04	0	0	0	0	na	na	0	na
Chicken breast, honey baked (Louis Rich)	1 slice	22.5	0.25/0	0	0	0	0	na	na	0	na
Chicken breast, roasted, fat-free (Oscar Mayer)	1 slice	11	0.08/0.02	0	0	0	0	na	na	0	na
Chicken breast, smoked, 97% fat-free (Louis Rich)	1 slice	30	1/0	0	0	0	0	na	na	na	na
Ham lunch meat, 98% fat-free (Healthy Favorites)	1 slice	12.5	0.25/0	0	0	0	0	na	na	na	na
Ham lunch meat, extra lean	1 slice	37	1.4/0.5	0	0	0	0	1	4.6	0	0.12

Food	Serving Size	Calories	Fat/Sat. Fat (gm)	Fiber (gm)	Flavonoids (mg)	Carotenoids (mcg or mg)	PE (mcg or mg)	Folate (mcg)	Selenium (mcg)	Vit. C (mg)	Vit. E (IUs)
Ham lunch meat, lowfat (Oscar Mayer)	1 slice	22	0.8/0.18	0	0	0	0	na	na	0	na
Lunch meat, light (Spam)	2 oz.	140	12/4	0	0	0	0	na	na	na	na
Turkey breast	1 slice	30	2/0	0	0	0	0	na	na	na	na
Turkey breast, 95% fat-free (Louis Rich)	1 slice	35	1/0	0	0	0	0	na	na	na	na
Turkey breast, roasted (Mr. Turkey)	1 slice	33	0.8/0.3	0	0	0	0	1	na	0.01	na
Turkey breast, smoked, fat-free (Oscar Mayer)	1 slice	10	0.08/0.02	0	0	0	0	na	0	na	na
Turkey ham (Louis Rich)	1 slice	15	0.4/0.1	0	0	0	0	na	na	0	na
Turkey ham, chopped (Louis Rich)	1 oz.	46	3/0.7	0	0	0	0	na	na	na	na
Turkey ham, honey-cured (Louis Rich)	1 slice	30	1/0	0	0	0	0	na	na	0	na
Turkey ham, smoked (Mr. Turkey)	1 slice	33	1.5/0.5	0	0	0	0	2	na	0.03	na
Turkey loaf, 89% fat-free (Louis Rich)	1 slice	45	3/0	0	0	0	0	na	na	na	na
Turkey pastrami (Mr. Turkey)	1 slice	31	1/0.3	0	0	0	0	1.4	na	0.01	na
Turkey salami (Louis Rich)	1 slice	40	2.5/1	0	0	0	0	na	na	0	na

Food	Serving Size	Calories	Fat/Sat. Fat (gm)	Fiber (gm)	Flavonoids (mg)	Carotenoids (mcg or mg)	PE (mcg or mg)	Folate (mcg)	Selenium (mcg)	Vit. C (mg)	Vit. E (IUs)
SAUSAGE, LEAN											
Pork, light	1 link	70	5/0	0	0	0	0	na	na	na	na
Smoked sausage, lowfat (Healthy Choice)	2 oz.	70	1.5/0.5	0	0	0	0	na	na	2.4	na
Turkey, brown & serve	1 link	40	2/0.6	0.1	0	0	0	4.6	4	0	0
Turkey, smoked	1 medium slice	56	4/1	0	0	0	0	2	3.6	0	0.15
Turkey, Polish (Mr. Turkey)	1 oz.	59	4/0	0	0	0	0	na	na	na	na
Turkey and pork	1 patty	77	6/2	0	0	0	0	1	5	0.3	0.15
Turkey, pork, and beef, lowfat	1 medium slice	58	1.4/0.5	0	0	0	0	3.4	14	1	0.15
Turkey, pork, and beef, reduced fat	1 medium slice	137	10/3.5	0	0	0	0	2.3	16	0	0.15
Turkey summer sausage (Louis Rich)	1-oz. slice	55	4/1	0	0	0	0	na	na	na	na
SNACKS/CHIPS											
Apple chips (Weight Watchers)	1 pouch	50	1/0	0	na	3 mcg (BC)	na	na	na	na	na
Banana chips	1 oz.	147	9.5/8	2	na	46 mcg (BC)	na	4	0.4	2	2.3
Brown rice chips	1 oz.	130	5/0	0	na	na	na	na	na	na	na
Carrot chips	1 oz.	150	9/0	0	na	1.7 mg (BC)	na	na	na	na	na

180

Food	Serving Size	Calories	Fat/Sat. Fat (gm)	Fiber (gm)	Flavonoids (mg)	Carotenoids (mcg or mg)	PE (mcg or mg)	Folate (mcg)	Selenium (mcg)	Vit. C (mg)	Vit. E (IUs)
Potato chips, baked	1 oz.	120	1/0	0	na	0	na	na	na	na	na
Potato chips, barbecue, baked	1 oz.	110	1.5/0	0.7	na	0	na	na	na	0	na
Potato chips, dietetic (Spicer's)	1 oz.	100	4/0	9	na	0	na	na	na	na	na
Potato chips, less fat (Ruffles)	1 oz.	130	6/1	1	na	0	na	na	na	na	na
Potato chips, light (Pringles)	1 oz.	150	8/0	0	na	0	na	na	na	na	na
Sea vegetable chips (Eden Foods)	1 oz.	130	5/0	0	na	na	na	na	na	na	na
Tortilla chips, lowfat	10 chips	44	0.5/0	0.5	na	52 mcg (BC)	na	na	na	na	na
Tortilla chips, nacho, baked	1 oz.	110	1/0	2	na	52 mcg (BC)	na	na	na	0	na
Tortilla chips, nacho, light	1 oz.	126	4/0.8	1.4	na	na	na	7	na	0.6	na
Tortilla chips, nacho cheese, light	1 oz.	120	4/0	0	na	na	na	na	na	na	na
Vegetable chips (Eden Foods)	1 oz.	130	4/0	0	na	na	na	na	na	na	na
SNACKS/CRISPS, CURLS, OR PUFFS											
Bagel crisps	1 oz.	130	4/1	1	0	na	na	na	na	na	na
Cheddar flavored puffs, light	1 oz.	120	4/1	na	0	na	na	na	na	0.6	na
Cheese flavored puffs, nonfat	1 cup	73	0/0	1.3	0	na	na	2.7	na	0	na

181

Food	Serving Size	Calories	Fat/Sat. Fat (gm)	Fiber (gm)	Flavonoids (mg)	Carotenoids (mcg or mg)	PE (mcg or mg)	Folate (mcg)	Selenium (mcg)	Vit. C (mg)	Vit. E (IUs)
Corn puffs, caramel, nonfat (Health Valley)	1 cup	110	0/0	2	0	na	na	4	na	0	na
Corn puffs, cheese (Ultra Slim-Fast)	1 oz.	110	3/0	3	0	na	na	na	na	na	na
SNACKS/FRUIT BARS AND SNACKS											
Apple fruit bar, nonfat (Health Valley)	1 bar	70	0/0	2	na	na	na	na	na	2.4	na
Apple raisin bar (Weight Watchers)	1 bar	70	2/0.5	2	na	na	na	na	na	0	na
Fruit roll, enriched (Sunkist)	1 roll	72	0.2/0	1.6	na	na	na	na	na	17	na
Fruit roll-up (Betty Crocker)	2 rolls	104	1/0.3	na	na	10 mcg (BC)	na	na	1	34	na
Fruit snack bar (Earth Grains)	1 bar	240	3/0	0	na	na	na	na	na	na	na
Yogurt-coated raising	9 pieces	170	7/5	1	na	na	na	na	na	na	na
SNACKS/GRAIN CAKES											
Corn cakes:											
Apple cinnamon	1	49	1/0	0	na	na	na	na	na	na	na
Butter flavor (Quaker)	1	35	0/0	0	na	na	na	na	na	na	na
Caramel flavor (Chico-San)	1	50	0/0	0	na	na	na	na	na	na	na

182

Food	Serving Size	Calories	Fat/Sat. Fat (gm)	Fiber (gm)	Flavonoids (mg)	Carotenoids (mcg or mg)	PE (mcg or mg)	Folate (mcg)	Selenium (mcg)	Vit. C (mg)	Vit. E (IUs)
Plain	1	35	0.2/0.04	0.2	na	3.6 mcg (BC)	na	2	1	0	0.02
White Cheddar (Roman Meal)	1	45	0/0	0	na	na	na	na	na	na	na
Rice cakes:											
Apple cinnamon	1	50	0/0	0	na	na	na	na	na	0	na
Brown rice, multigrain	1	35	0.3/0.05	0.3	na	0	na	2	na	0	na
Brown rice, plain	1	35	0.25/0.05	0.4	na	0	na	2	2	0	0.1
Brown rice, rye	1	35	0.35/0.05	0.4	na	0	na	0.5	na	0	na
Brown rice, sesame seed	1	35	0.35/0.05	0.5	na	0	na	1.6	2	0.3	na
Corn (Quaker)	1	35	0.2/0	0.2	na	3.6 mcg (BC)	na	na	na	na	na
Rice, 5-grain (Hain)	1	40	1/0	0	na	na	na	na	na	na	na
Rice, plain	1	40	1/0	0	na	0	na	na	na	na	na
Rice, rye (Quaker)	1	35	0.3/0	0.8	na	na	na	na	na	na	na
Rice, sesame (Hain)	1	40	1/0	0	na	na	na	na	na	na	na
Rice, wheat (Quaker)	1	34	0.3/0.1	0.8	na	na	na	na	na	na	na
SNACKS/POPCORN											
Butter flavored (Pop Secret— Betty Crocker)	3 cups	70	3/0	2	na	na	na	na	na	na	na
Cracker Jacks	½ cup	120	2/0	1	na	7.5 mcg (BC)	na	na	na	0	na
Microwave (Jolly Time)	3 cups	120	7/1.5	3	na	na	na	na	na	na	na

Food	Serving Size	Calories	Fat/Sat. Fat (gm)	Fiber (gm)	Flavonoids (mg)	Carotenoids (mcg or mg)	PE (mcg or mg)	Folate (mcg)	Selenium (mcg)	Vit. C (mg)	Vit. E (IUs)
Microwave, light— (Pop Secret— Betty Crocker)	3 cups	70	3/1	2	na	na	na	na	na	na	na
Natural flavor (Healthy Choice)	3 cups	45	0/0	1.5	na	na	na	na	na	0	na
Popped, white "Gourmet" (Orville Redenbacher)	3 cups	80	4/0	3	na	na	na	na	na	na	na
Popped, air, white	3 cups	92	3/0.14	3.6	na	29 mcg (BC)	na	5.5	2.4	0	na
Popped, air, yellow (Jolly Time)	3 cups	60	1/0	4	na	29 mcg (BC)	na	na	na	na	na
White cheddar flavored (Weight Watchers)	1 pkg.	100	6/0	0	na	77 mcg (BC)	na	na	na	na	na
SNACKS/PRETZELS											
Multi-grain, nonfat	30 pretzels	110	0/0	3	na	na	na	na	na	0	na
9-grain	2 pretzels	100	1.5/0	3	na	na	na	na	na	12	na
Nonfat	16 pretzels	100	0/0	1	na	na	na	na	na	0.6	na
Oat bran	1 oz.	115	1.5/0	0.3	na	na	na	na	na	na	na
Plain	10 pretzels	229	2/0.5	1.7	na	0	na	50	0	3.5	na
Rice bran	1 oz.	101	2/0	2	na	na	na	na	na	na	na
Sesame, chips (Nabisco)	8 chips	60	2/0	0	na	0	na	na	na	0	na
Soft	1 pretzel	190	0/0	2	na	na	na	na	na	na	na
Sticks, thin, lowfat	1 oz.	110	3/0	1	na	na	na	na	na	na	na

Food	Serving Size	Calories	Fat/Sat. Fat (gm)	Fiber (gm)	Flavonoids (mg)	Carotenoids (mcg or mg)	PE (mcg or mg)	Folate (mcg)	Selenium (mcg)	Vit. C (mg)	Vit. E (IUs)
Sticks, nonfat	47 sticks	110	0/0	1	na	na	na	na	na	0.6	na
Yogurt coated	⅓ cup	140	5/4	0	na	na	na	na	na	na	na
SNACKS/SNACK MIXES											
Fruit and nut (Planter's)	1 oz.	150	10/3	t	na	na	na	na	na	na	na
Party mix, lowfat	1 oz.	120	1.5/0	1	na	na	na	na	na	1.2	na
Snack mix	½ cup	150	7/1	1	na	22.5 mcg (BC)	na	na	na	0	na
Snack mix, baked (Ritz)	1 oz.	130	6/1	0	na	na	na	na	na	na	na
Snack mix, barbecued (Chex—Ralston)	1 oz.	130	5/0	0	na	na	na	na	na	na	na
Snack mix, nonfat	¾ cup	120	0/0	1	na	na	na	na	na	na	na
Snack mix, w/ nuts (Pepperidge Farm)	½ cup	180	9/1.5	2	na	na	na	na	na	na	na
Snack mix, oriental	1 oz.	156	7/1	4	na	na	na	11	2.3	0.09	3.6
Trail mix, regular	½ cup	347	22/4	na	na	5.4 mcg (BC)	na	53	na	1	na
Trail mix, tropical	½ cup	285	12/6	na	na	na	56 mg	29	na	5	na
SOUPS/CONDENSED (PREPARED WITH WATER UNLESS OTHERWISE SPECIFIED)											
Asparagus, prep. w/ milk	1 cup	161	8/3	0.75	na	285 mcg (BC)	na	30	na	4	1.26
Bean w/ pork	1 cup	172	6/1.5	9	na	532 mcg (BC)	na	32	8	1.5	0.11
Beef broth	1 cup	60	0/0	0	0	0	0	6	5	1.7	na
Beef & mushroom	1 cup	73	3/1.5	0.25	na	3 mg (BC)	na	10	na	4.6	na
Beef noodle	1 cup	83	3/1	0.7	0	376 mcg (BC)	na	19.5	7	0.25	t

Food	Serving Size	Calories	Fat/Sat. Fat (gm)	Fiber (gm)	Flavonoids (mg)	Carotenoids (mcg or mg)	PE (mcg or mg)	Folate (mcg)	Selenium (mcg)	Vit. C (mg)	Vit. E (IUs)
Black bean	1 cup	116	1.5/0.4	4.5	na	296 mcg (BC)	na	25	1	0.7	0.11
Broccoli cheese, prep. w/ milk	1 cup	165	9/3.4	2	na	500 mcg (BC)	na	27	4	3.4	2.5
Celery	1 cup	90	5.6/1.4	0.7	na	180 mcg (BC)	na	2.5	2	0.25	1.35
Cheese	1 cup	156	10.5/7	1	na	670 mcg (BC)	na	5	4.5	0	na
Chicken broth	1 cup	38	1.4/0.4	0	na	0	0	5	0	0	0.06
Chicken gumbo	1 cup	56	1.5/0.3	2	na	88 mcg (BC)	na	5	8	5	0.06
Chicken mushroom	1 cup	132	9/2.4	0.25	na	693 mcg (BC)	na	0.25	6	na	na
Chicken noodle	1 cup	75	2.5/0.65	0.7	na	993 mcg (BC)	na	22	6	0.25	0.1
Chicken vegetable	1 cup	75	3/0.8	1	na	1.5 mg (BC)	na	5	5	1	0.12
Chicken w/ dumplings	1 cup	96	5.5/1.3	0.5	na	309 mcg (BC)	na	2.4	12	0	0.2
Chicken w/ rice	1 cup	60	2/0.5	0.7	na	990 mcg (BC)	na	1	5	0.24	0.08
Chili beef	1 cup	170	6.6/3.3	9.5	na	900 mcg (BC)	na	17.5	6	4	0.26
Clam chowder, Manhattan	1 cup	78	2/0.4	1.5	na	828 mcg (BC)	na	10	9	4	0.6
Clam chowder, New England, prep. w/ milk	1 cup	164	6.6/3	1.5	na	14 mcg (BC)	na	9.7	13	3.5	0.22
Minestrone	1 cup	82	2.5/0.5	1	na	1.4 mg (BC) 3.7 mg (LYC)	na	36	na	1.2	0.1
Mushroom, cream of, prep. w/ milk	1 cup	203	13.6/5	0.5	na	14 mcg (BC)	na	10	4	2.2	2
Mushroom barley	1 cup	73	2.3/0.4	0.7	na	3 mcg (BC)	na	5	na	0	na
Onion	1 cup	58	2/0.26	1	na	0	na	15	4	1.2	0.43
Oyster stew, prep. w/ milk	1 cup	135	8/5	0	na	67 mcg (BC)	na	10	na	4.4	na

186

Food	Serving Size	Calories	Fat/Sat. Fat (gm)	Fiber (gm)	Flavonoids (mg)	Carotenoids (mcg or mg)[b]	PE (mcg or mg)	Folate (mcg)	Selenium (mcg)	Vit. C (mg)	Vit. E (IUs)
Pea, prep. w/ milk	1 cup	239	7/4	3	na	132 mcg (BC)	na	8	na	3	0.27
Pea, split w/ Ham	1 cup	190	4.4/1.7	2.3	na	1.3 mg (BC)	na	2.5	na	1.5	na
Pepperpot	1 cup	104	4.6/2	0.5	na	521 mcg (BC)	na	10	4	1.5	0.13
Potato, prep. w/ milk	1 cup	149	6.5/4	0.5	na	187 mcg (BC)	na	9	4	1.2	0.15
Shrimp, prep. w/ milk	1 cup	90	5/3	0.25	0	113 mcg (BC)	na	3.7	5.6	0	1.2
Tomato, prep. w/ milk	1 cup	161	6/3	3	na	436 mcg (BC) 27 mg (LYC)	na	21	2	68	4
Tomato beef	1 cup	139	4.3/1.6	1.5	na	322 mcg (BC)	na	19.5	5	0	1.2
Tomato bisque, prep. w/ milk	1 cup	198	6.6/3	0.5	na	436 mcg (BC)	na	21	7	7	na
Tomato rice	1 cup	119	3/0.5	1.5	na	712 mcg (BC)	na	13.5	2	15	1.2
Turkey	1 cup	68	2/0.6	0.7	0	na	na	19.5	11	2.5	0.09
Turkey noodle	1 cup	69	2/0.6	0.8	na	173 mcg (BC)	na	19	11	0.1	0.15
Turkey vegetable	1 cup	72	3/1	0.5	na	1.3 mg (BC)	na	5	na	0	0.2
Vegetable beef	1 cup	78	2/0.8	0.5	na	1 mg (BC) 9 mg (LYC)	na	10.5	4.4	2.5	0.5
Vegetable beef broth	1 cup	82	2/0.4	0.5	na	na	na	9.6	2.7	2.4	0.5
SOUPS/DRY MIX (PREPARED WITH WATER UNLESS OTHERWISE SPECIFIED)											
Asparagus	1 cup	58	1.7/0.05	na	na	271 mcg (BC)	na	7.5	na	0.75	na
Bean w/ bacon	1 cup	106	2/1	9	na	532 mcg (BC)	na	8	6	1	0.4
Beef noodle	1 cup	40	0.8/0.25	0.75	na	376 mcg (BC)	na	15	4.5	0.5	0.04
Beefy mushroom (Lipton)	1 serving	33	0.4/0.05	0.11	na	0	na	0	na	0.16	na
Beefy onion (Lipton)	1 serving	25	0.6/0.14	0.35	na	na	na	0	na	0.65	na

Food	Serving Size	Calories	Fat/Sat. Fat (gm)	Fiber (gm)	Flavonoids (mg)	Carotenoids (mcg or mg)	PE (mcg or mg)	Folate (mcg)	Selenium (mcg)	Vit. C (mg)	Vit. E (IUs)
Broccoli & cheese (Lipton Cup-a-Soup)	1 serving	67	3/0.8	0.7	na	na	na	3.7	na	3	na
Cauliflower	1 cup	69	1.7/0.25	na	na	109 mcg (BC)	na	2.6	na	2.5	na
Celery, cream of	1 cup	63.5	1.6/0.25	na	na	180 mcg (BC)	na	1	na	0.25	na
Chicken	1 cup	106	5/3	0.5	0	434 mcg (BC)	0	5.4	na	0.5	0.2
Chicken broth, fat-free (Lipton Cup-a-Soup)	1 serving	18	0.13/0.02	t	na	0	na	0	na	0.02	na
Chicken noodle	1 cup	55	1.3/0.3	0.24	na	2 mcg (BC)	na	17	9	0	0.13
Chicken pasta, fat-free (Lipton Cup-a-Soup)	1 serving	44	0.3/0.5	0.15	na	na	na	14	na	0.06	na
Chicken rice	1 cup	58	1.4/0.3	0.7	na	716 mcg (BC)	na	0.5	5	0	0.04
Chicken supreme (Lipton Cup-a-Soup)	1 serving	90	3.75/1.4	0.65	na	na	na	0	na	0.13	0
Chicken vegetable	1 cup	50	0.8/0.17	na	na	na	na	2.5	4	1.25	na
Clam chowder, Manhattan	1 cup	65	1.5/0.26	na	na	828 mcg (BC)	na	10	na	4	na
Clam chowder, New England	1 cup	95	3.7/0.6	1	na	0	na	3	na	2	2
Consommé	1 cup	17	0.02/0	0	0	0	0	4	2	0	0
Green pea (Lipton Cup-a-Soup)	1 serving	75	1/0.2	3	na	32 mcg (BC)	na	0	na	0.04	na
Herb, fiesta (Lipton)	1 serving	29	0.3/0.05	0.4	na	na	na	2	na	1.5	na
Leek	1 cup	71	2/1	3	na	0	na	7.6	5	2.5	0.23
Lentil (Lipton Homestyle)	1 serving	127	1/0.1	5	na	1 mg (BC)	na	29	na	1	na
Minestrone	1 cup	79	2/0.8	na	na	na	na	35	3.5	1	na

Food	Serving Size	Calories	Fat/Sat. Fat (gm)	Fiber (gm)	Flavenoids (mg)	Carotenoids (mcg or mg)	PE (mcg or mg)	Folate (mcg)	Selenium (mcg)	Vit. C (mg)	Vit. E (IUs)
Mushroom (Lipton Cup-a-Soup)	1 serving	60	2/0.3	0.5	na	0	na	0	na	0.12	na
Mushroom	1 cup	96	5/0.8	0.8	na	0	na	5	5	1	na
Noodle rings (Lipton Cup-A-Soup)	1 serving	53	1/0.4	0.2	na	na	na	17	na	0.15	na
Onion	1 cup	27	0.5/0.12	1	na	0	na	1.5	2.5	0.25	0.15
Onion mushroom	1 serving	32	0.8/0.1	0.32	na	na	na	0	na	0.5	na
Oxtail	1 cup	68	2.5/1	0.5	na	0	na	5	2	0	0.1
Pasta & bean (Lipton Homestyle)	1 serving	125	1.4/0.3	4	na	181 mcg (BC)	na	46	na	2	na
Pasta, spirals (Lipton)	1 serving	64	1/0.3	0.4	na	na	na	24.5	na	0.05	na
Pea	1 cup	133	1.6/0.4	3	na	32 mcg (BC)	na	42	5	0	0.2
Potato	1 cup	68	0.6/0.1	1.5	na	0	na	7	2.5	3	0.15
Ramen noodle (Nissin)	1 serving	190	7/3	na	na	0	na	na	na	na	na
Savory herb w/ garlic (Lipton)	1 serving	31	0.4/0.09	0.3	na	na	na	0	na	1.7	na
Tomato	1 cup	103	2.4/1	0.5	na	493 mcg (BC)	na	6.6	0.5	4.5	1.3
Tomato vegetable	1 cup	53	0.8/0.4	0.5	na	116 mcg (BC)	na	9.6	4	6	1.15
Vegetable, cream of	1 cup	105	5.7/1.4	0.7	na	638 mcg (BC)	na	7	5	4	2
Vegetable beef	1 cup	53	1/0.5	0.5	na	1 mg (BC)	na	7.6	3	1.3	0.04
Vegetable (Lipton Cup-a-Soup)	1 serving	52	1/0.35	0.3	na	137 mcg (BC)	na	13	na	0.5	na

Food	Serving Size	Calories	Fat/Sat. Fat (gm)	Fiber (gm)	Flavonoids (mg)	Carotenoids (mcg or mg)	PE (mcg or mg)	Folate (mcg)	Selenium (mcg)	Vit. C (mg)	Vit. E (IUs)
Vegetable, spring (Lipton Cup-a-Soup)	1 serving	47	1/0.2	0.65	na	na	na	13.5	na	0.6	na
SOUPS/READY-TO-SERVE											
Bean, home recipe	1 cup	140	0.4/0.1	7	na	4 mg (BC)	na	73	2	5	0.6
Bean, mixed (inc. 15-bean soup)	1 cup	130	1.5/0.4	6	na	137 mcg (BC)	na	92	6	6	0.6
Bean w/ ham, chunky	1 cup	231	8.5/3.3	11	na	3 mg (BC)	na	29	17	4.4	na
Beef barley, lowfat (Progresso Healthy Classics)	1 cup	137	1.7/0.7	3.6	na	na	na	na	na	na	na
Beef barley (Progresso Healthy Classics)	1 cup	142	2/0.75	3	na	3 mcg (BC)	na	24	na	3.6	0.4
Beef soup, chunky	1 cup	170	5/2.5	1.5	na	na	na	13.5	6	7	0.25
Beef stew (Dinty Moore)	1 cup	222	13/6	2.6	na	4.2 mg (BC)	na	na	na	2.6	na
Beef stew (Nestle's Chef Mate)	1 cup	191.5	6/2.4	3.3	na	na	na	na	na	2.5	0.84
Beef vegetable, chunky (Campbell's)	1 cup	153	4.4/1.3	na	na	1.5 mg (BC)	na	na	na	na	na
Beef vegetable w/ rice, chunky	1 cup	181	5/2.4	1.4	na	1.5 mg (BC)	na	22	7	6.4	0.3
Beef soup, milk-based	1 cup	109	3.6/1.4	0.6	na	6 mcg (BC)	na	21	10	0.5	0.45

190

Food	Serving Size	Calories	Fat/Sat. Fat (gm)	Fiber (gm)	Flavonoids (mg)	Carotenoids (mcg or mg)	PE (mcg or mg)	Folate (mcg)	Selenium (mcg)	Vit. C (mg)	Vit. E (IUs)
Beet (borscht)	1 cup	78.5	4/2.3	2	na	6 mcg (BC)	na	47	2	9	0.45
Broccoli (Progresso Healthy Classics)	1 cup	88	2.8/0.7	2.4	na	53 mcg (BC)	na	29	na	6	0.57
Carrot, milk-based	1 cup	60	1.6/0.6	1.3	na	5.3 mg (BC)	na	11	1	1.4	0.3
Carrot and rice, milk-based	1 cup	88.5	1.5/0.6	1.3	na	4.9 mg (BC)	na	25	3	1.3	0.3
Cauliflower, milk-based	1 cup	197	12/4	1.5	na	109 mcg (BC)	na	36	6	23	2
Chicken, chunky	1 cup	170	6/2	1.4	na	773 mcg (BC)	na	4	na	1	0.25
Chicken corn chowder, chunky	1 cup	238	15/4	2	na	na	na	na	na	na	na
Chicken mushroom chowder, chunky	1 cup	192	11/2.7	3.3	na	na	na	na	na	5	na
Chicken noodle (Progresso Healthy Classics)	1 cup	76	1.6/0.4	1	na	1.4 mg (BC)	na	33	na	0.7	0.1
Chicken rice, chunky (Campbell's)	1 cup	127	3/1	1	na	3.5 mg (BC)	na	4	11	4	0.13
Chicken vegetable, chunky	1 cup	166	5/1.4	1	na	4 mg (BC)	na	12	12	5.5	na
Chicken vegetable w/ potatoes & cheese, chunky	1 cup	175	12/4.4	0.8	na	194 mcg (BC)	na	8	10	11	1.65
Chicken w/ wild rice (Progresso)	1 cup	93	2/0.6	na	na	na	na	na	na	na	na
Chili beef	1 cup	192	7/3	4.5	na	128 mcg (BC)	na	83	9	7	0.3

Food	Serving Size	Calories	Fat/Sat. Fat (gm)	Fiber (gm)	Flavonoids (mg)	Carotenoids (mcg or mg)	PE (mcg or mg)	Folate (mcg)	Selenium (mcg)	Vit. C (mg)	Vit. E (IUs)
Chili con carne w/ beans	1 cup	255	8/2	8	na	719 mcg (BC)	na	57	5	0.88	0.4
Chili con carne w/o beans	1 serving	305	20/7.5	3.7	na	976 mcg (BC)	na	na	na	na	na
Chili w/ beans (Hormel)	1 cup	240	4.4/1.8	8.4	na	na	na	na	na	0.5	na
Chili w/ beans (Nestlé's Chef Mate)	1 cup	412	25/11	11	na	na	na	na	na	0.8	1.8
Chili w/ beans (Old El Paso)	1 serving	248	10/2	10	na	na	na	na	na	na	na
Chili w/ beans, spicy (Nestlé's Chef Mate)	1 cup	422.5	25/11	4	na	na	na	na	na	1.27	3
Chili w/ beans, vegetarian (Hormel)	1 cup	205	0.7/0.12	10	na	na	na	na	na	1.2	na
Chili w/o beans (Hormel)	1 cup	193.5	6.6/2	3	na	na	na	na	na	0	na
Chili w/o beans (Nestlé's Chef Mate)	1 cup	430	32/14	3	na	na	na	na	na	1.75	2.3
Clam chowder, Manhattan, chunky	1 cup	134	3.4/2	3	na	828 mcg (BC)	na	9	16	12	0.14
Clam chowder, New England, chunky (Progresso Healthy Classics)	1 cup	117	2/0.5	1	na	5 mcg (BC)	na	29	na	5	0.8
Crab	1 cup	76	1.5/0.4	0.7	na	77 mcg (BC)	na	15	6	0	na
Cucumber, milk-based	1 cup	197.5	12/4	0.5	na	155 mcg (BC)	na	18	6	3	2
Duck	1 cup	410	37/12.5	0.3	0	t	0	16	20	3.6	0.75
Egg drop	1 cup	73	4/1	0	0		0	15	7.5	0	0.45
Escarole	1 cup	28	2/0.5	na	na	843 mcg (BC)	na	35	na	4.5	na

Food	Serving Size	Calories	Fat/Sat. Fat (gm)	Fiber (gm)	Flavonoids (mg)	Carotenoids (mcg or mg)	PE (mcg or mg)	Folate (mcg)	Selenium (mcg)	Vit. C (mg)	Vit. E (IUs)
Fruit soup	1 cup	176	0.2/0	4	na	504 mcg (BC)	na	0.4	0.8	2	0.45
Garbanzo	1 cup	207	3/0.3	9	na	19 mcg (BC)	na	106	5.5	2	0.6
Garlic egg	1 cup	180.5	11/2	0.4	na	0	na	31	17	0	1.65
Garlic & pasta (Progresso Healthy Classics)	1 cup	100	1.3/0.3	3	na	na	na	63	10	0	0.4
Gazpacho	1 cup	46	0.25/t	0.5	na	1.5 mg (BC)	na	10	3.7	7	0.7
Leek, cream of, milk-based	1 cup	172	8/3	0.5	na	195 mcg (BC)	na	12	5.5	2	1.35
Lentil (Progresso Healthy Classics)	1 cup	126	1.5/0.3	6	na	1 mg (BC)	na	102	na	1	0.9
Lentil w/ ham	1 cup	139	3/1	na	na	1 mg (BC)	na	50	0.75	4	na
Lima bean	1 cup	111	3/1	5	na	2.5 mg (BC)	na	51	2	3.4	0.6
Macaroni and potato	1 cup	211	3.3/1.4	3	na	23 mcg (BC)	na	32	6	20	0.6
Matzo ball	1 cup	119	5.5/1.3	0.4	na	0	na	19	6	0	1
Minestrone (Progresso Healthy Classics)	1 cup	123	2.5/0.4	1	na	1.2 mg (BC)	na	60	na	0.7	0.6
Minestrone, chunky	1 cup	127	3/1.5	6	na	na	na	53	5	5	0.6
Onion, cream of, milk-based	1 cup	172	8/3	0.5	na	195 mcg (BC)	na	12	5.5	2	1.35
Onion, French	1 cup	58	2/0.3	1	na	0	na	15	4	1	0.45
Pea, split (Progresso Healthy Classics)	1 cup	180	2.3/0.76	5	na	1.3 mg (BC)	na	51	0.8	0	0.5
Pean, split w/ ham, chunky	1 cup	185	4/1.6	4	na	3 mg (BC)	na	4.6	10	7	2
Pea, split w/ ham, chunky, reduced fat	1 cup	185	2.6/0.7	na	na	na	na	na	na	10	na

Food	Serving Size	Calories	Fat/Sat. Fat (gm)	Fiber (gm)	Flavonoids (mg)	Carotenoids (mcg or mg)	PE (mcg or mg)	Folate (mcg)	Selenium (mcg)	Vit. C (mg)	Vit. E (IUs)
Pinto bean	1 cup	191	0.7/0.1	**13**	na	0	na	**132**	10.5	3	0.15
Potato cheese	1 cup	187	8/4.6	1	na	44 mcg (BC)	na	18.5	6	10	0.6
Potato chowder, chunky	1 cup	192	12.5/4	1.5	na	46 mcg (BC)	na	83	5	na	1.35
Seaweed	1 cup	83	4/1	0.6	na	125 mcg (BC)	0	19.5	na	3	10
Shark fin	1 cup	99	4/1	0	0	na	0	na	na	0.2	na
Sirloin burger vegetable (Campbell's)	1 cup	185	9/3	**5.5**	na	**1.5 mg (BC)**	na	na	na	na	na
Spinach	1 cup	204	12/4	2	na	**3.6 mg (BC)**	na	**105**	7	8	2.85
Sweet and sour	1 cup	72	0.8/0.3	1.6	na	187 mcg (BC)	na	16	5	17	0.75
Tomato garden (Progresso Healthy Classics)	1 cup	99	1/0.17	4	na	na	na	25	4.4	5	0.9
Tortilla	1 cup	238	14/4	1.4	na	106 mcg (BC)	na	62	11	6.6	2
Turkey, chunky	1 cup	134.5	4.4/1	na	na	na	na	12	na	6.4	na
Turkey noodle, chunky	1 cup	177	5/1.4	1.3	na	**1.8 mg (BC)**	na	36.5	**29**	0.9	0.45
Turtle and vegetable	1 cup	118	4/0.8	0.7	na	98 mcg (BC)	na	18.5	12	7	1.35
Vegetable (Progresso Healthy Classics)	1 cup	81	1.3/0.3	1.5	na	1 mg (BC)	na	29	na	1.5	0.2
Vegetable beef	1 cup	128.5	2/0.65	4.4	na	1 mg (BC)	na	na	7	na	0.9
Vegetable, chunky	1 cup	122	4/0.5	1	na	**3.2 mg (BC)**	na	17	2	6	0.9
Vegetable, home recipe	1 cup	100	4.5/0.9	2	na	**1.3 mg (BC)**	na	60	5	12	1.65
Vichyssoise	1 cup	136	5/3	0.5	na	187 mcg (BC)	na	9	9	1	0.3
White bean	1 cup	242	7/2.3	4	na	1.5 mcg (BC)	na	79	9	11	0.6

Food	Serving Size	Calories	Fat/Sat. Fat (gm)	Fiber (gm)	Flavonoids (mg)	Carotenoids (mcg or mg)	PE (mcg or mg)	Folate (mcg)	Selenium (mcg)	Vit. C (mg)	Vit. E (IUs)
Wonton	1 cup	182	7/2.3	0.9	na	na	na	33.5	18	3	0.6
Zucchini, cream of, milk-based	1 cup	169	10/3	1	na	203 mcg (BC)	na	25	5	5	1.8
SOY FOODS & PRODUCTS											
Natto	2 tsp.	19	1/0.1	0.5	na	0	5 mg	0.7	0.8	1.2	0
Nutlettes breakfast cereal	½ cup	140	1.5/na	9	na	na	122 mg	na	na	na	0
Miso	½ cup	284	8/1.2	7	na	74 mcg (BC)	15 mg	46	2.2	0	0
Miso broth	1 cup	85	3.4/0.6	2	na	2.7 mg (BC)	na	57	0.8	4.4	1
Soybeans, cooked from dry	1 cup	311	16/2.3	11	na	11 mcg (BC)	220 mg	97	13	3	5
Soybeans, dry roasted, (soy nuts)	½ cup	219	12/1.7	8	na	56 mcg (BC)	470 mcg (L) 128–167 mg	98	9	1	1
Soy bacon	1 strip	16	1.5/0.2	0.1	na	3 mcg (BC)	t	2.1	0.4	0	0.45
Soy buffalo wings (Morningstar Farms)	5 pieces	200	9/1.5	3	na	na	na	na	na	na	na
Soy burgers/patties: Generic	1 patty	140	6.3/1	3.2	na	0	na	na	0.6	0	1.8
Better'n burgers (Morningstar Farms)	1 patty	80	0/0	3	na	na	na	na	na	0	na
Breakfast patties (Morningstar Farms)	1 patty	80	3/0.5	2	na	na	na	na	na	0	na

Food	Serving Size	Calories	Fat/Sat. Fat (gm)	Fiber (gm)	Flavonoids (mg)	Carotenoids (mcg or mg)	PE (mcg or mg)	Folate (mcg)	Selenium (mcg)	Vit. C (mg)	Vit. E (IUs)
Harvest burger (Morningstar Farms)	1 patty	140	4/1.5	5	na	na	7.4 mg	na	na	na	na
Soybean butter	2 tbsp.	170	11.6/t	0.3	na	na	17 mg	na	na	na	na
Soybean butter, roasted (Natural Touch, Morningstar Farms)	2 tbsp.	170	11/1.5	1	na	na	17 mg	na	na	0	na
Soy cheeses:											
Unspecified	1 oz.	80–110	0–7/t	0	na	na	9 mg	na	na	na	4.5
Cheddar	1 oz.	40	3/na	0	na	na	2 mg	na	na	na	na
Mozzarella	1 oz.	20	0/0	0	na	na	2 mg	na	na	na	na
Soybean curd cheese	4 oz.	151	9/1.3	0	na	27 mcg (BC)	32 mg	25	19	0	0.7
Soybean chips (GeniSoy Crisps)	25 pieces	100	2/0	2	na	na	5 mg	na	na	0	na
Soy cookies (EssenSmart):											
Almond Delight	1 ea.	136	4/t	1.2	na	na	26 mg	na	na	na	na
Orange & Raisin	1 ea.	126	2/0	1.4	na	na	33 mg	na	na	na	na
Ginger & Spice	1 ea.	136	4/t	1.4	na	na	34 mg	na	na	na	na

SOY FOODS & PRODUCTS/SOY BEVERAGES

Food	Serving Size	Calories	Fat/Sat. Fat (gm)	Fiber (gm)	Flavonoids (mg)	Carotenoids (mcg or mg)	PE (mcg or mg)	Folate (mcg)	Selenium (mcg)	Vit. C (mg)	Vit. E (IUs)
GeniSoy Natural Protein Powder	1 scoop	100	0/0	0	na	na	74 mg	100	50	15	45
GeniSoy Shake—chocolate	1 scoop	120	0/0	2	na	na	na	100	50	15	45
GeniSoy Shake—vanilla	1 scoop	130	0/0	0	na	na	na	100	50	15	45

Food	Serving Size	Calories	Fat/Sat. Fat (gm)	Fiber (gm)	Flavonoids (mg)	Carotenoids (mcg or mg)	PE (mcg or mg)	Folate (mcg)	Selenium (mcg)	Vit. C (mg)	Vit. E (IUs)
Revival:											
Chocolate Daydream, w/ fructose	1 packet	240	2.5/1	2	na	na	160 mg	na	na	na	na
Chocolate Daydream, unsweetened	1 packet	130	2.5/1	0	na	na	160 mg	na	na	na	na
Slim-Fast Chocolate Delite w/ soy protein	2 scoops	170	2/1	1	na	na	na	200	17.5	60	45
SoyaMax	2 scoops	106	1.2/na	na	na	na	60 mg	na	na	na	na
Spirutein Shake—cappuccino	2 scoops	100	0/0	na	na	na	16 mg	400	21	60	45
Spirutein Shake—chocolate	2 scoops	99	0/0	na	na	na	15 mg	400	21	60	45
Super-Green Pro-96	2 scoops	100	1/0	0	na	12 mcg (BC)	27 mg	na	na	1.2	na
Ultra Slim-Fast w/ soy protein	1 can	220	1/0	5	na	na	na	200	17.5	60	45
SOY FOODS & PRODUCTS											
Soy bread	1 slice	69	1/3	0.9	na	na	na	23	5.4	0.1	0.15
Soy flour	¼ cup	94	5/na	2	na	na	100 mg	48	na	na	na
Soy flour, defatted	¼ cup	82	0.3/na	4.4	na	na	73 mg	76	na	na	na
Soy grits, dry	¼ cup	140	6/1	6	na	na	na	na	na	na	na
Soy hot dog	1 ea.	62–140	1.5–7/1.1	3.2	na	0	8.5–35 mg	55	5	0	2
Big Franks (Loma Linda)	1 ea.	110	7/1	2	na	na	2 mg	na	na	0	na

Food	Serving Size	Calories	Fat/Sat. Fat (gm)	Fiber (gm)	Flavonoids (mg)	Carotenoids (mcg or mg)	PE (mcg or mg)	Folate (mcg)	Selenium (mcg)	Vit. C (mg)	Vit. E (IUs)
Soy luncheon meat	1 reg. slice	78	4.5/0.7	1.4	na	0	na	28	2	0	1
Soy links (Morningstar Farms)	2 links	60	2/0.5	2	na	na	20–30 mg	na	3.2	0	na
Soy milk	1 cup	81–140	4.7/0.5	3.2	na	44 mcg (BC)	na	4	na	0	0
Soy milk, lowfat	1 cup	100	2/t	na	na	na	na	na	na	na	na
Edensoy Original Extra	1 cup	130	4/0.5	0	na	na	na	40	na	na	11
Edensoy Original	1 cup	130	5/0.5	0	na	na	41 mg	40	na	na	na
WestSoy:											
100% Organic Original	1 cup	100	4.5/0.5	4	na	na	na	na	na	0	na
100% Organic Original Plain	1 cup	140	4.5/0	3	na	na	na	na	na	0	na
Lite Cocoa	1 cup	120	1.5/0	2	na	na	na	na	na	0	na
Lite Plain	1 cup	90	2/0	2	na	na	na	na	na	0	na
Lite Vanilla	1 cup	120	2.5/0.5	3	na	na	na	na	na	0	na
Low Fat Chocolate	1 cup	180	3/0	3	na	na	na	na	na	0	na
Low Fat Plain	1 cup	110	1.5/0	2	na	na	na	na	na	0	na
Low Fat Vanilla	1 cup	110	1.5/0	2	na	na	na	na	na	0	na
Soy noodles	1 cup	500	0.1/0	5.5	na	0	18 mg	0	38	0	0
Soy nuggets	1 cup	286	20/3	7.4	na	0	20 mg	94	12.4	0	5
Soy protein, textured	¼ cup	80	0/0	4	na	na	28 mg	na	na	na	0
Soy sauce, regular	1 tbsp.	8.5	0/0	0.1	na	0	na	2.5	0.1	0	0
Soy sauce, reduced sodium	1 tbsp.	8.5	0/0	0.1	na	0	na	2.5	0.1	0	0

Food	Serving Size	Calories	Fat/Sat. Fat (gm)	Fiber (gm)	Flavonoids (mg)	Carotenoids (mcg or mg)	PE (mcg or mg)	Folate (mcg)	Selenium (mcg)	Vit. C (mg)	Vit. E (IUs)
Soy sprouts	1 cup	100	6/na	2	na	na	na	na	na	na	na
Soy supplement bars:											
GeniSoy Apple Spice Bar	1 bar	220	4/3	1	na	na	33mg	100	50	15	45
GeniSoy Chocolate Bar	1 bar	220	3.5/2.5	1	na	na	33 mg	100	50	15	45
High-protein bar, soy-based	1 bar	325	13.5/2	1.9	na	1.3 mg (BC)	na	116	0	27	2
Soy yogurt	1 cup	102–150	2–4/na	1	na	na	20–25 mg	na	na	na	na
Tempeh	½ cup	165	6.4/na	7	na	na	35–53 mg	28	na	0	na
Tempeh burger	1 patty	245	7.4/na	0.9	na	na	29–32 mg	na	na	0.1	na
Tofu, regular	½ cup	94	6/0.9	1	na	67 mcg (BC)	24–38 mg	41	11	0.1	0
Tofu, firm	½ cup	97–120	6/1	1	na	67 mcg (BC)	25 mg	42	11	0.1	0
Tofu, silken	½ cup	72	2.4/t	0	na	67 mcg (BC)	29 mg	42	11	0.1	0
Tofu, soft	½ cup	86	5/1	0	na	67 mcg (BC)	25 mg	42	11	0.1	0
Tofutti, chocolate	1 cup	359	24/5.2	6	na	11 mcg (BC)	33 mg	12	4	0	5
Tofutti, flavors other than chocolate	1 cup	427	30/4	1.2	na	19 mcg (BC)	33 mg	22	2.3	0.5	6
TOMATOES AND TOMATO PRODUCTS											
Canned, chopped	½ cup	30	0/0	2	na	11.25 mg (LYC)	na	9	0.8	18	0.75
Canned, crushed	½ cup	29	0.25/0	1.5	na	11.25 mg (LYC)	na	9	0.8	11	0.75
Canned, whole	½ cup	25	0/0	1	na	11.5 mg (LYC)	na	9	0.8	17	0.75
Fresh, boiled	½ cup	32	0.5/0.07	1.3	na	360 mcg (BC) 5 mg (LYC)	11 mg	16	0.6	27	na

Food	Serving Size	Calories	Fat/Sat. Fat (gm)	Fiber (gm)	Flavonoids (mg)	Carotenoids (mcg or mg)	PE (mcg or mg)	Folate (mcg)	Selenium (mcg)	Vit. C (mg)	Vit. E (IUs)
Marinara sauce	½ cup	71	2.6/0.4	2	na	285 mcg (BC) 20 mg (LYC)	na	12.5	0.75	10	2.4
Marinara sauce (Contadina)	½ cup	80	4/0.5	2	na	na	na	na	na	na	na
Marinara sauce (Prego)	½ cup	110	6/1.5	3	na	na	na	na	na	18	na
Paste	½ cup	107	0.7/0.1	5.4	na	1.6 mg (BC) 38 mg (LYC)	na	29	2	56	8.5
Pizza sauce (Contadina)	½ cup	34	0.7/0.3	1.3	na	na	na	6	na	7	2.4
Puree	½ cup	50	0.2/0.02	2.5	na	512 mcg (BC) 21 mg (LYC)	na	13	1	13	5
Raw, cherry	1 cherry	4	0.06/t	0.2	na	na	na	2.5	0.07	3.3	0.1
Raw, green	1 medium	30	0.25/0.03	1.4	na	na	na	11	0.5	29	0.7
Raw, Italian	1 medium	13	0.2/0.02	0.7	na	na	4.3 mg	9	0.25	12	0.35
Raw, orange	1 medium	18	0.2/0.03	1	na	na	4.4 mg	32	0.5	18	na
Raw, red	1 medium	26	0.4/0.05	1.4	na	483 mcg (BC) 3.7 mg (LYC)	9 mg	18.5	0.5	24	0.7
Raw, yellow	1 medium	32	0.6/0.07	1.5	55 mg	na	13 mg	64	1	19	na
Sauce, canned	½ cup	90	3/1	1	na	512 mcg (BC) 22 mg (LYC)	na	11.5	0.75	16	2.5
Spaghetti sauce:											
chunky	½ cup	50	1/0	2	na	na	na	na	na	na	na
Garlic (Healthy Choice)	½ cu	40	0/0	0	na	na	na	na	na	na	na
Herb (Ragú)	½ cup	50	1/0	0	na	na	na	na	na	na	na
Homestyle (Hunt's)	½ cup	60	2/0.3	2	na	na	na	na	na	na	na

Food	Serving Size	Calories	Fat/Sat. Fat (gm)	Fiber (gm)	Flavonoids (mg)	Carotenoids (mcg or mg)	PE (mcg or mg)	Folate (mcg)	Selenium (mcg)	Vit. C (mg)	Vit. E (IUs)
Italian (Healthy Choice)	½ cup	40	0/0	0	na	na	na	na	na	na	na
Meat (Contadina)	½ cup	100	3/1	0	na	na	na	1.4	na	11	na
Meat (Prego)	½ cup	140	6/1.5	3	na	na	na	na	na	12	na
Meat (Ragú)	½ cup	110	5/0	3	na	na	na	na	na	na	na
Meatless	½ cup	48	1/0.16	na	na	na	na	na	na	4	na
Mushroom (Healthy Choice)	½ cup	50	0.7/0	2.3	na	285 mcg (BC)	na	na	na	10	na
Mushroom (Prego)	½ cup	110	3/1	3	na	285 mcg (BC)	na	na	na	9	na
Mushroom (Ragú)	½ cup	110	3/0	0	na	285 mcg (BC)	na	na	na	9	na
Parmesan	½ cup	50	2/0.3	2	na	na	na	na	na	5	na
Plain	½ cup	140	4.5/1.5	2	na	285 mcg (BC) 20 mg (LYC)	na	na	na	9	na
Ready to serve	½ cup	70	1.6/0.19	2.4	na	285 mcg (BC) 20 mg (LYC)	na	12.5	na	11	4.7
Sausage	½ cup	180	9/2.5	3	na	na	na	na	na	21	na
Tomato and basil	½ cup	110	3/0.5	3	na	na	na	na	na	21	na
Vegetable (Hunt's)	½ cup	62	1/0.1	2	na	na	na	na	na	29	na
Vegetable (Healthy Choice)	½ cup	50	0.6/0	2.5	na	na	na	na	na	8	na
Stewed	½ cup	35	0/0	2	na	na	na	6.6	0.8	15	0.75
Sundried	½ cup	70	0.8/0.1	3.3	na	na	na	18.5	1.5	10.5	0
TURKEY											
Roasted:											
Breast (meat/skin)	100 gm	189	7.4/2	0	0	0	0	6	29	0	0

Food	Serving Size	Calories	Fat/Sat. Fat (gm)	Fiber (gm)	Flavonoids (mg)	Carotenoids (mcg or mg)	PE (mcg or mg)	Folate (mcg)	Selenium (mcg)	Vit. C (mg)	Vit. E (IUs)
Dark meat	1 cup	262	10/3.4	0	0	0	0	12.6	57	0	0.9
Leg	1 leg	148	7/2	0	0	0	0	6.4	27	0	1.4
Light meat	1 cup	276	12/3	0	0	0	0	8.4	41	0	0
Giblets, simmered	1 cup	242	7/2	0	0	0	0	500	322	2.5	3
Patty:											
Breaded, fried	1 patty (2.25 oz.)	181	11.5/3	0.3	0	0	0	18	13	0	2
Cooked	1 patty (4 oz.)	193	11/3	0	0	0	0	6	30.5	0	0.4

TURKEY PRODUCTS

Food	Serving Size	Calories	Fat/Sat. Fat (gm)	Fiber (gm)	Flavonoids (mg)	Carotenoids (mcg or mg)	PE (mcg or mg)	Folate (mcg)	Selenium (mcg)	Vit. C (mg)	Vit. E (IUs)
Turkey ham (Louis Rich)	1 deli-thin slice	15	0.38/0.12	0	0	0	0	0	0	0	0
Turkey ham, honey cured (Louis Rich)	1 slice	30	1/0	0	0	0	0	0	0	0	0
Turkey ham, smoked (Mr. Turkey)	1 oz.	32	1.3/0	0	0	0	0	0	0	0	0

VEAL

Food	Serving Size	Calories	Fat/Sat. Fat (gm)	Fiber (gm)	Flavonoids (mg)	Carotenoids (mcg or mg)	PE (mcg or mg)	Folate (mcg)	Selenium (mcg)	Vit. C (mg)	Vit. E (IUs)
Blade, roasted	3 oz.	158	7/3	0	0	0	0	9	9	0	0.6
Chop, broiled	1 medium chop	232	13/5.6	0	0	0	0	16	12	0	0.75
Cutlet, broiled	1 cutlet	136	4/1.6	0	0	0	0	13.6	9.5	0	0.6
Cutlet, breaded, fried	1 cutlet	194	8/2.6	0.3	0	0	0	23	14	0	0.75

Food	Serving Size	Calories	Fat/Sat. Fat (gm)	Fiber (gm)	Flavonoids (mg)	Carotenoids (mcg or mg)	PE (mcg or mg)	Folate (mcg)	Selenium (mcg)	Vit. C (mg)	Vit. E (IUs)
Ground, broiled	3 oz.	146	6.4/2.5	0	0	0	0	9	12	0	0.2
Liver, pan-fried	3 oz.	208	9.6/3.5	0	0	0	0	272	45	19	0.6
VEGETABLES & LEGUMES											
Alfalfa sprouts, raw	1 cup	10	0.2/0.02	1	na	na	na	12	0.2	3	t
Artichoke:											
Hearts, canned in water	⅔ cup	44	0/0	6	na	na	na	45	na	7	0.3
Hearts, cooked from frozen	3 oz.	30	0/0	4	na	na	na	95	na	4	0.2
Marinated	½ cup	168	14/2	8	na	na	na	149	na	52	3
Whole artichoke, globe, cooked	1 medium	60	0.2/0.04	6.5	na	na	na	61	0.24	12	0.35
Arugula, raw, chopped	1 cup	5	0.1/t	0.3	na	na	na	20	0.06	3	0.1
Asparagus, cooked:											
Canned spears	6 spears	21	0.7/0.2	2	na	na	na	103	2	20	0.7
From fresh, cuts and tips	½ cup	22	0.3/0.06	1.5	na	na	22 mg	131	1.5	10	0.5
From fresh, spears	6 spears	22	t/t	2	na	na	na	131	na	10	0.5
From frozen, cuts and tips	½ cup	25	0.4/0.1	1.5	na	na	na	121	1.5	22	na
From frozen, spears	6 spears	25	t/t	2	na	na	na	122	na	10	0.5
Bamboo shoots, canned, drained slices	1 cup	15	0.3/0.06	1	na	na	na	3	0.5	1	0.75
Beans, cooked:											
Adzuki, boiled	½ cup	147	0.1/0.04	8	na	na	na	139	1.5	0	na

203

Food	Serving Size	Calories	Fat/Sat. Fat (gm)	Fiber (gm)	Flavonoids (mg)	Carotenoids (mcg or mg)	PE (mcg or mg)	Folate (mcg)	Selenium (mcg)	Vit. C (mg)	Vit. E (IUs)
Black beans, canned	½ cup	114	0.4/0.1	7.5	na	na	na	128	1	0	na
Black-eyed peas	½ cup										
Chickpeas (garbanzo), canned	½ cup	135	2/0.2	7	na	na	na	141	3	1	na
Fava, canned	½ cup	91	0.2/0.04	5	na	na	na	42	2.5	2.5	na
Great northern, canned	½ cup	149	0.5/0.1	7	na	na	na	107	5	2	na
Kidney, boiled	½ cup	113	0.4/0.06	7	na	na	na	115	1	1	na
Kidney, canned	½ cup	104	0.4/0.05	4.5	na	na	na	63	1.5	1.5	na
Lima, boiled	½ cup	105	0.25/0.05	5	na	na	na	23	2	8	na
Lima, canned	½ cup	88	0.4/0.08	5	na	na	na	20	1.5	9	0.5
Lima, cooked from frozen	½ cup	85	0.3/0.06	5	na	na	na	18	1.5	11	na
Mung, boiled	½ cup	106	0.3/0.1	8	na	na	na	160	2.5	1	na
Navy, boiled	½ cup	129	0.5/0.1	6	na	na	na	127	5	1	na
Navy, canned	½ cup	148	0.5/0.1	7	na	na	na	82	7.5	1	0.7
Pinto, boiled	½ cup	117	0.4/0.09	7	na	na	na	147	6	2	na
Pinto, canned	½ cup	103	1/0.2	5.5	na	na	na	72	9	1	1.7
Snap, green string and French style:											
Canned	½ cup	18	0.1/0.03	2	na	na	na	22	0.3	4	0.2
From fresh	½ cup	22	0.1/0.04	2	na	na	na	21	0.3	6	0.1
From frozen	½ cup	18	0.1/0.03	2	na	na	na	15	0.25	3	0.15
Snap, yellow:											
Canned	½ cup	18	0.1/0.03	2	na	na	na	22	0.25	4	na

Food	Serving Size	Calories	Fat/Sat. Fat (gm)	Fiber (gm)	Flavonoids (mg)	Carotenoids (mcg or mg)	PE (mcg or mg)	Folate (mcg)	Selenium (mcg)	Vit. C (mg)	Vit. E (IUs)
From fresh	½ cup	22	0.1/0.04	2	na	na	na	21	0.25	6	0.3
From frozen	½ cup	18	0.1/0.02	2	na	na	na	15	0.25	3	0.3
White, boiled	½ cup	125	0.3/0.08	5.5	na	na	na	72	1	0	na
White, canned	½ cup	153	0.4/0.1	7	na	na	na	86	2	0	na
Bean sprouts (mung), raw	1 cup	31	0.2/0.05	2	na	na	16 mg	63	0.6	14	0.02
Bean sprouts (mung), canned	1 cup	15	0.08/0.02	1	na	na	na	12	0.8	0.4	0.02
Beets:											
Raw	2 beets	70	0.3/0.04	5	na	na	41 mg	179	1	8	0.8
Canned, sliced	½ cup	26	0.1/0.02	1.5	na	na	na	25	0.4	3.5	0.4
Cooked from fresh, sliced	½ cup	37	0.15/0.02	2	na	na	na	68	0.6	3	na
Pickled slices	½ cup	74	0.09/0.01	3	na	na	na	30	1	2.5	na
Whole, canned	1 cup	51	0.3/0.03	3	na	na	na	49	0.8	7	0.7
Whole, cooked from fresh	2 beets	44	0.2/0.03	3	na	na	na	80	0.7	4	0.5
Beet greens, cooked	½ cup	20	0.14/0.02	2	na	1.8 mg(BC)	na	10	0.7	18	na
Breadfruit, cooked	½ cup	145	0.3/0.1	7	na	31 mcg (BC)	na	13	0.8	31	2.4
Broccoli, raw:											
Chopped	1 cup	25	0.3/0.05	2.6	2.6	685 mcg (BC) 2 mg (LU+Z)	na	63	2.6	82	2
Spears	2	18	0.05/t	2	1.9	483 mcg (BC) 1.5 mg (LU+Z)	na	44	2	58	1.5

Food	Serving Size	Calories	Fat/Sat. Fat (gm)	Fiber (gm)	Flavonoids (mg)	Carotenoids (mcg or mg)	PE (mcg or mg)	Folate (mcg)	Selenium (mcg)	Vit. C (mg)	Vit. E (IUs)
Broccoli, cooked from fresh:											
Chopped	½ cup	22	0.3/0.04	2	2	813 mcg (BC) 1.7 mg (LU+Z)	na	39	1.5	58	2
Spears	2	21	0.3/0.04	2	2	771 mcg (BC) 1.6 mg (LU+Z)	na	37	1.4	55	2
Broccoli, cooked from frozen:											
Chopped	½ cup	25	0.1/0.01	2	2.8	920 mcg (BC) 764 mcg (LU+Z)	na	52	5.5	37	4.5
Spears	½ cup	26	0.1/0.01	3	2.8	920 mcg (BC) 764 mcg (LU+Z)	na	28	2	37	1.4
Broccoli sprouts											
Broccoflower:											
Raw	1 cup	20	0.2/0	2	na	58 mcg (BC)	na	37	0.4	56	0
Cooked	½ cup	14	0.1/0	1.5	na	37 mcg (BC)	na	18	0.3	32	0
Brussels sprouts:											
Cooked from fresh	½ cup	32	0.4/0.08	2	na	363 mcg (BC) 1 mg (LU+Z)	na	47	1	48	1
Cooked from frozen	½ cup	33	0.3/0.02	3	na	na	na	78	1	36	0.7
Cabbage, common varieties:											
Raw, shredded, or chopped	1 cup	22	0.2/0.03	2	na	58 mcg (BC) 276 mcg (LU+Z)	10 mg	38	0.8	29	0.14
Cooked, drained	½ cup	17	0.3/0.04	2	na	68 mcg (BC)	na	15	0.5	15	0.12

Food	Serving Size	Calories	Fat/Sat. Fat (gm)	Fiber (gm)	Flavonoids (mg)	Carotenoids (mcg or mg)	PE (mcg or mg)	Folate (mcg)	Selenium (mcg)	Vit. C (mg)	Vit. E (IUs)
Cabbage:											
Bok choy, raw, shredded	1 cup	9	0.1/0.01	0.7	na	na	na	46	0.4	32	0.13
Bok choy, cooked	½ cup	10	0.1/0.01	1.5	na	na	na	35	0.3	22	0.15
Cabbage, red:											
Raw, chopped	1 cup	19	0.2/0.02	1.4	na	na	na	15	0.6	40	0.1
Cooked, drained	½ cup	16	0.15/0.02	1.5	na	na	na	10	0.5	26	na
Cabbage, savoy:											
Raw, chopped	1 cup	19	0.07/t	2	na	na	na	56	0.6	22	0.1
Cooked, drained	½ cup	17	0.05/t	2	na	na	na	34	0.5	13	na
Capers	1 tbsp.	2	0.07/0.02	0.3	na	7 mcg (BC)	4 mg	2	0.1	0.4	0.1
Carrots:											
Fresh, grated	1 cup	47	0.2/0.03	3	na	5 mg (AC) 9.7 mg (BC)	13 mg	15	1	10	0.75
Fresh, whole	1 medium	26	0.1/0.02	2	na	2.8 mg (AC) 5.4 mg (BC)	7 mg	8.5	0.7	6	0.4
Carrots, sliced:											
Canned	½ cup	28	0.2/0.03	2	na	4.3 mg (AC) 7 mg (BC)	na	10	0.5	2.5	0.7
Cooked from fresh, drained	½ cup	35	0.1/0.02	2.5	na	3.2 mg (AC) 6.3 mg (BC)	na	11	0.6	2	0.5
Cooked from frozen, drained	½ cup	26	0.08/0.01	2.5	na	4 mg (AC) 9 mg (BC)	na	8	0.4	2	0.45

Food	Serving Size	Calories	Fat/Sat. Fat (gm)	Fiber (gm)	Flavonoids (mg)	Carotenoids (mcg or mg)	PE (mcg or mg)	Folate (mcg)	Selenium (mcg)	Vit. C (mg)	Vit. E (IUs)
Carrots, baby:											
Raw	4 medium	15	0.2/0.04	0.7	na	1.7 mg (AC) 3 mg (BC)	na	13	0.4	3	na
Cooked from frozen	2/3 cup	35	0/0	2	na	na	na	na	na	1	na
Cauliflower:											
Raw	1 cup	25	0.2/0.03	2.5	na	na	18 mg	57	0.6	46	0.06
Cooked from fresh, drained	½ cup	14	0.3/0.04	2	na	na	na	27	0.3	27	0.04
Cooked from frozen, drained	½ cup	17	0.2/0.03	2.5	na	na	na	37	1	28	0.1
Celery:											
Raw	1 medium stalk	6	0.06/0.02	0.7	na	60 mcg (AC) 93 mcg (LU+Z)	2.4 mg	11	0.4	3	0.2
Cooked from fresh	½ cup	13	0.1/0.03	1	na	158 mcg (BC) 188 mcg (LU+Z)	5 mg	16	0.75	4.5	0.4
Celeriac root, cooked	½ cup	21	0.15/0	0.5	na	na	na	2.5	0.3	2.5	na
Chard, Swiss:											
Raw	1 cup	7	0.6/0.01	0.6	na	1.4 mg (BC)	na	5	0.3	11	1
Cooked from fresh	½ cup	17	0.07/0	2	na	na	na	7.5	0.75	16	na
Chayote:											
Raw	1 chayote	39	0.3/0.06	3.5	na	0	na	189	0.4	16	0.4
Cooked	½ cup	19	0.3/0.07	2	na	na	na	15	0.2	7	na

Food	Serving Size	Calories	Fat/Sat. Fat (gm)	Fiber (gm)	Flavonoids (mg)	Carotenoids (mcg or mg)	PE (mcg or mg)	Folate (mcg)	Selenium (mcg)	Vit. C (mg)	Vit. E (IUs)
Collards:											
Cooked from fresh	½ cup	25	0.3/0.04	2.5	na	4 mg (BC)	na	88	1	18	1
Cooked from frozen	½ cup	30	0.35/0.05	2.5	na	7.7 mg (LU+Z)	na	65	1	23	0.6
Corn (white):											
Canned	½ cup	66	0.8/0.1	1.5	na	na	na	40	0.5	7	0.1
Cooked from fresh, cob	1 ear	59	0.5/0.07	2	na	na	na	19	0.4	3	na
Cooked from frozen, cob	1 ear	68	0.4/0.1	2	na	0	na	26	0.6	3	0.15
Cream style	½ cup	92	0.5/0.08	1.5	na	na	na	57	0.8	6	0.2
Kernels, cooked from frozen	½ cup	89	1/0.2	2	na	na	na	38	0.7	5	0.1
Corn (yellow):											
Canned	½ cup	83	0.5/0.08	2	na	928 mcg (LU+Z)	na	52	0.7	8.5	0.14
Cooked from fresh, cob	1 ear	83	1/0.15	2	na	1.4 mg (LU+Z)	na	36	0.6	5	na
Cooked from frozen, cob	1 ear	68	0.4/0.1	2	na	43 mcg (BC)	na	26	0.6	3	0.15
Cream style	½ cup	92	0.5/0.08	1.5	na	na	na	57	0.75	6	0.2
Kernels, cooked from frozen	½ cup	82	0.6/0.09	2	na	64 mcg (BC)	na	49	0.8	7	na
Cucumber slices w/ peel	1 cup	14	0.1/0.02	0.8	na	143 mcg (BC)	14 mg	14	0	6	0.1
Cucumber slices w/o peel	1 cup	14	0.2/0.05	1	na	37 mcg (BC)	na	17	0	3	0.1
Dandelion greens:											
Raw	1 cup	25	0.4/0.09	2	na	4.6 mg (BC)	na	15	0.3	19	2

209

Food	Serving Size	Calories	Fat/Sat. Fat (gm)	Fiber (gm)	Flavonoids (mg)	Carotenoids (mcg or mg)	PE (mcg or mg)	Folate (mcg)	Selenium (mcg)	Vit. C (mg)	Vit. E (IUs)
Cooked	½ cup	17	0.3/0.07	1.5	na	3.7 mg (BC)	na	6.5	0.15	9.5	2
Eggplant:											
boiled	1 cup	28	0.2/0.04	2.5	na	na	na	14	0.4	1.3	0.05
cubed, raw	1 cup	21	0.15/0.03	2	na	na	6 mg	16	0.25	1.4	0.04
Endive, fresh, chopped	1 cup	8.5	0.1/0.02	1.5	na	480 mcg (BC)	na	71	0.1	3	0.3
Grape leaves, raw	1 cup	13	0.3/0.05	1.5	na	2.3 mg (BC)	3 mg	12	0.1	1.5	0.4
Jicama, raw	1 cup	49	0.1/0.03	6	na	na	na	16	0.9	26	0.9
Kale:											
Raw, chopped	1 cup	34	0.5/0.06	1	7	6 mg (BC) 26 mg (LU+Z)	na	20	0.6	80	0.8
Cooked from fresh	½ cup	19.5	0.3/0.04	1	7	4 mg (BC) 10 mg (LU+Z)	na	9.5	0.5	16	0.7
Cooked from frozen	½ cup	19.5	0.3/t	1	7	2.5 mg (BC)	na	9	0.6	16	0.15
Kohlrabi:											
Raw	1 cup	36	0.1/0.01	5	na	na	na	22	1	84	1
Cooked	½ cup	24	0.09/t	1	na	na	na	10	0.7	45	1
Leeks:											
Raw	1 leek, bulb/ lower leaves	54	0.3/0.04	1.6	t	na	na	57	1	11	1
Cooked	1 leek, bulb/ lower leaves	38	0.2/0.03	1	t	na	na	30	0.6	5	na
Lentils:											
Cooked from dry	½ cup	115	0.3/0.05	8	na	na	na	179	3	1.5	0.2
Sprouted	1 cup	82	0.4/0.04	3	na	na	na	77	0.5	13	0.3

210

Food	Serving Size	Calories	Fat/Sat. Fat (gm)	Fiber (gm)	Flavonoids (mg)	Carotenoids (mcg or mg)	PE (mcg or mg)	Folate (mcg)	Selenium (mcg)	Vit. C (mg)	Vit. E (IUs)
Lettuce, raw, chopped:											
Boston/butterhead	1 cup	7	0.1/0.01	0.6	1	na	na	40	0.1	4	0.4
Escarole	1 cup	8	t/t	1	na	na	na	71	na	3	0.3
Iceberg	1 cup	7	0.1/0.01	0.8	1	106 mcg (BC); 194 mcg (LU+Z)	6 mg	31	0.1	2	0.2
Looseleaf	1 cup	10	0.2/0.02	1	1	na	21 mg	28	0.1	10	0.4
Radicchio	1 cup	9	0.1/0.02	0.4	na	na	na	24	0.4	3	1.4
Romaine	1 cup	8	t/t	1	na	712 mcg (BC); 1.5 mg (LU+Z)	na	38	na	7	0.2
Mushrooms:											
Raw, common types, sliced	1 cup	18	0.2/0.03	0.9	na	na	na	8	6	1.6	0.13
Canned, common types	½ cup, pieces	19	0.2/0.03	2	na	na	na	10	3	0	0.14
Caps, pickled	8	11	t/t	1	na	na	na	6	na	1	0.08
Cooked from raw	½ cup, pieces	21	0.4/0.05	2	na	na	na	14	9	3	0.14
Oyster, raw	1 large	55	0.8/0	4	na	na	na	70	27	0	na
Portobello, raw	3½ oz.	26	0.2/0.03	1.5	na	na	na	22	11	0	0.2
Shiitake, cooked	½ cup, pieces	40	0.2/0.04	1.5	na	na	na	15	18	0.2	0.13
Shiitake, dried	4 mushrooms	44	0.15/0.04	2	na	na	na	25	20	0.5	0.03
Straw, canned	½ cup	29	0.6/0.08	2	na	0	na	35	14	0	na

Food	Serving Size	Calories	Fat/Sat. Fat (gm)	Fiber (gm)	Flavonoids (mg)	Carotenoids (mcg or mg)	PE (mcg or mg)	Folate (mcg)	Selenium (mcg)	Vit. C (mg)	Vit. E (IUs)
Okra:											
Raw	1 cup	33	0.1/0.03	3	na	28 mcg (AC) 432 mcg (BC)	24 mg	88	0.7	21	1
Cooked from fresh, sliced	½ cup	26	0.1/0.04	2	na	136 mcg (BC) 312 mcg (LU+Z)	na	37	0.6	13	0.8
Cooked from frozen, sliced	½ cup	34	0.1/t	3	na	na	na	na	na	11	0.1
Onions:											
Raw	1 medium	42	0.2/0.03	2	38	na	17 mg	21	0.7	7	0.2
Raw, chopped	½ cup	31	0.1/0.02	1.5	28	na	12 mg	15	0.5	5	0.16
Cooked	½ cup	46	0.2/0.03	1.5	36	na	19 mg	16	0.5	5.5	0.2
Green, spring, chopped	½ cup, bulb/top	16	t/t	1	na	196 mcg (BC)	na	32	na	9	0.1
Flakes, dehydrated	1 tbsp.	17	t/t	0.5	na	na	na	8	0.25	4	0.1
Palm hearts, canned	1 cup	41	1/0.2	3.5	na	na	na	57	1	12	na
Parsley, raw:											
Chopped	½ cup	11	0.2/0.03	1	na	1 mg (BC)	1.5 mg	46	0.06	40	0.75
Sprigs	5	2	t/t	0.1	na	156 mcg (BC)	t	7.5	t	6.5	0.1
Parsnips, cooked, sliced	½ cup	63	0.2/0.04	3	na	na	na	45	1	10	na
Peas:											
Green, canned	½ cup	59	0.3/0.05	3.5	na	272 mcg (BC)	na	38	1.5	8	0.5
Green, cooked from fresh	½ cup	62	0.2/0.04	4	na	1 mg (LU+Z)	na	47	0.8	8	0.2

212

Food	Serving Size	Calories	Fat/Sat. Fat (gm)	Fiber (gm)	Flavonoids (mg)	Carotenoids (mcg or mg)	PE (mcg or mg)	Folate (mcg)	Selenium (mcg)	Vit. C (mg)	Vit. E (IUs)
Green, cooked from frozen	½ cup	62	0.2/0.04	4	na	256 mcg (BC)	na	47	0.8	8	0.2
Pod peas, edible, cooked	½ cup	33	t/t	2	na	na	na	24	na	38	0.5
Split peas, cooked from dry	½ cup	115	0.4/0.05	8	na	na	na	63	0.5	0.4	0.6
Peppers:											
Banana, raw	1 medium	12	0.2/0.02	1.5	na	18 mcg (AC) 85 mcg (BC)	1.4 mg	13	0.14	38	0.5
Chili, green, canned	½ cup	14	0.07/t	1	na	na	na	7	0.2	46	0.7
Chili, green, raw	1 medium	18	0.09/t	0.7	na	na	na	11	0.2	109	0.5
Chili, red, canned	½ cup	14	0.07/t	1	na	na	na	7	0.2	46	0.7
Chili, red, raw	1 medium	18	0.09/t	0.7	na	na	na	11	0.2	109	0.5
Jalapeño, sliced, canned	½ cup	14	0.5/0.05	3	na	na	na	8	0.2	5	0.36
Jalapeño, raw	1 medium	18	0.1/0	0.7	na	1.5 mg (BC)	na	11	0.2	109	0.45
Peppers, sweet, green:											
Raw	1 medium	32	0.2/0.03	2	na	635 mcg (BC)	11 mg	26	0.4	106	1
Cooked, chopped	½ cup	19	0.1/0.02	0.8	na	na	6 mg	11	0.2	51	0.7
Peppers, sweet, red:											
Raw	1 medium	32	0.2/0.03	0.2	na	70 mcg (AC) 2.8 mg (BC)	11 mg	26	0.4	226	1
Cooked, chopped	½ cup	19	0.1/0.02	0.8	na	42 mcg (AC) 1.5 mg (BC)	6 mg	11	0.2	116	0.7
Marinated	1 oz.	10	0/0	t	na	na	na	na	na	15	na

213

Food	Serving Size	Calories	Fat/Sat. Fat (gm)	Fiber (gm)	Flavonoids (mg)	Carotenoids (mcg or mg)	PE (mcg or mg)	Folate (mcg)	Selenium (mcg)	Vit. C (mg)	Vit. E (IUs)
Peppers, sweet, yellow:											
Raw	1 large	50	0.4/0.06	2	na	223 mcg (BC)	na	48	0.6	341	na
Strips	10 strips	14	0.1/0.02	0.5	na	62 mcg (BC)	na	14	0.2	95	na
Potatoes:											
Au gratin	1 cup	323	19/12	4	na	na	na	27	7	24	na
Baked w/ skin	1 medium	220	t/t	5	28	0	na	22	1.6	26	0.15
Baked w/o skin	1 medium	145	t/t	2	22	0	na	14	0.5	20	0.09
Boiled w/o skin	1 medium	116	t/t	2	25	0	na	12	na	10	0.1
Canned	1 cup	108	0.4/0.1	4	na	0	na	10	1.6	9	0.15
French fried from frozen	10 fries	100	4/0.6	2	na	na	na	6	0.2	5	0.1
Hash browns from frozen	½ cup	170	9/4	2	na	na	na	12	0.2	5	0.2
Mashed w/ whole milk	1 cup	162	1.3/0.7	4	na	0	na	17	1.3	14	0.15
Microwaved w/ skin	1 medium	212	t/t	5	na	0	na	24	1.6	30	0.15
Scalloped (Stouffer's)	½ cup	140	6/1	2	na	na	na	na	na	5	na
Pumpkin, mashed:											
Canned	½ cup	41	0.03/0.01	3.5	na	6 mg (AC) 8.5 mg (BC)	na	15	0.5	5	2
Cooked from fresh	½ cup	25	0.08/0.04	1.5	na	na	na	10.5	0.25	6	2
Radishes, raw	½ cup	12	0.3/0.02	1	na	na	4 mg	16	0.4	13	t
Rutabaga, cooked, mashed	½ cup	47	0.3/0.04	2	na	na	na	18	0.9	23	na
Sauerkraut, canned	1 cup	27	0.2/0.05	4	na	na	na	34	0.9	21	0.2
Seaweed, kelp, raw	2 tbsp.	4	0.06/0.03	0.13	na	na	na	18	0.07	0.3	0.13
Shallots, raw	1 tbsp.	7	0.01/t	t	na	na	0.5 mg	3.5	0.1	0.8	na

Food	Serving Size	Calories	Fat/Sat. Fat (gm)	Fiber (gm)	Flavonoids (mg)	Carotenoids (mcg or mg)	PE (mcg or mg)	Folate (mcg)	Selenium (mcg)	Vit. C (mg)	Vit. E (IUs)
Spinach:											
Raw	1 cup	7	0.1/0.02	1	na	1.7 mg (BC) 3.5 mg (LU+Z)	3 mg	58	0.3	8.5	0.9
Canned	½ cup	25	0.5/0.08	2.5	na	5 mg (BC)	na	105	1.5	15	2
Cooked from fresh	½ cup	20	0.25/0.03	2	na	4.7 mg (BC) 6.3 mg (LU+Z)	na	131	1.5	9	1.3
Cooked from frozen	½ cup	27	0.2/0.03	3	na	na	na	102	1.6	6	na
Squash, summer:											
Yellow, raw	1 cup	23	0.2/0.05	2	na	102 mcg (BC) 261 mcg (LU+Z)	na	29	0.2	17	0.2
Yellow, cooked	½ cup	14	0.07/0.1	1.5	na	na	na	11	0.2	3	0.2
Zucchini, raw	1 cup	17	0.2/0.04	1.5	na	508 mcg (BC) 2.6 mg (LU+Z)	na	27	0.25	11	0.2
Zucchini, cooked	½ cup	14	0.04/t	1.2	na	na	na	15	0.4	4	0.2
Squash, winter:											
Acorn, mashed	½ cup	41	0.1/0.03	3	na	600 mcg (BC)	na	14	0.5	8	na
Butternut, mashed	½ cup	47	0.08/0.01	3	na	1.3 mg (AC) 5.5 mg (BC)	na	20	0.5	4	na
Hubbard, mashed	½ cup	35	0.4/0.1	3.5	na	na	na	11	0.3	7.5	0.2
Spaghetti, baked or boiled	1 cup	42	0.4/0.1	2	na	na	na	12	0.5	5.5	na
Sweet potato:											
Baked in skin	1 medium	117	0.1/0.03	3.5	na	11 mg (BC)	na	26	0.8	28	0.5

Food	Serving Size	Calories	Fat/Sat. Fat (gm)	Fiber (gm)	Flavonoids (mg)	Carotenoids (mcg or mg)	PE (mcg or mg)	Folate (mcg)	Selenium (mcg)	Vit. C (mg)	Vit. E (IUs)
Canned, pieces	1 cup	344	1/0.02	6	na	31 mg (BC)	na	36	2.3	56	1.4
Mashed	1 cup	182	0.4/0.09	3.6	na	17 mg (BC)	na	33	1.4	53	0.75
Taro shoots, cooked slices	½ cup	10	0.05/0.01	na	na	na	na	1.5	0.5	13	na
Tomatillos:											
Raw	1 medium	11	0.4/0.05	0.7	na	na	na	2.4	0.2	4	0.2
Raw, chopped	1 cup	42	1/0.2	2.5	na	na	na	10	0.6	16	0.75
Turnips, cooked, mashed	1 cup	48	0.2/0.02	5	1.6	na	na	21	1.4	27	0.1
Turnip greens:											
Cooked from fresh	½ cup	25	0.3/0.08	3	na	3.7 mg (BC) 7 mg (LU+Z)	na	33	1	18	3.6
Cooked from frozen	½ cup	25	0.4/0.08	3	na	na	na	32	1	18	na
Water chestnuts:											
Canned, slices	½ cup	35	0.04/0.01	2	na	na	na	4	0.5	1	0.5
Canned, whole	4	14	0.02/t	0.7	na	na	na	2	0.2	0.4	0.2
Watercress, raw, chopped	1 cup	4	0.03/t	0.5	na	na	na	3	0.3	15	0.5
VEGETABLES & LEGUMES, MIXED											
Broccoli, corn, and red pepper	½ cup	60	1/0	3	na	na	na	na	na	na	na
Brussels sprouts, cauliflower, and carrots (Birds Eye)	½ cup	40	0/0	4	na	na	na	na	na	na	na
Cauliflower, zucchini, carrots, red pepper	½ cup	30	0/0	2	na	na	na	na	na	na	na

Food	Serving Size	Calories	Fat/Sat. Fat (gm)	Fiber (gm)	Flavonoids (mg)	Carotenoids (mcg or mg)	PE (mcg or mg)	Folate (mcg)	Selenium (mcg)	Vit. C (mg)	Vit. E (IUs)
Corn w/ peppers (Mexican corn)	½ cup	89	1/0.2	2	na	136 mcg (BC)	na	39	7	11	0.15
Green beans and almonds	½ cup	97	7/0.7	2	na	190 mcg (BC)	na	20	0.8	5	4
Green beans and onions	½ cup	23	0.1/0	2	na	138 mcg (BC)	na	16	0.3	3	0.15
Green beans and potatoes	½ cup	41	0.1/0	2	na	143 mcg (BC)	na	15	0.2	6	0.15
Green beans and tomatoes	½ cup	25	0.2/0	2	na	347 mcg (BC)	na	18	0.3	8	0.6
Mixed vegetables, canned	½ cup	43	0.2/0	3	na	6 mg (BC)	na	20	0.3	4	0.75
Mixed vegetables, from frozen	½ cup	54	0.1/0	4	na	2.3 mg (BC)	na	17	0.3	3	0.45
Mixed vegetables, from frozen California blend (Freshlike)	½ cup	30	0/0	t	na	na	na	na	na	na	na
Mixed vegetables, from frozen, Italian blend (Freshlike)	½ cup	30	0/0	t	na	na	na	na	na	na	na
Oriental-style mixed vegetables	½ cup	24	0.1/0	2	na	348 mcg (BC)	na	20	2	na	1
Peas and carrots, canned	½ cup	50	0/0	t	na	na	na	na	na	na	na
Peas and carrots, from frozen	½ cup	60	1/0	t	na	na	na	na	na	na	na
Peas and corn	½ cup	78	0.6/0.1	3	na	198 mcg (BC)	na	44	1	8	0.3
Peas and mushrooms	½ cup	54	0.2/0	4	na	258 mcg (BC)	na	41	3	7	0.15

Food	Serving Size	Calories	Fat/Sat. Fat (gm)	Fiber (gm)	Flavonoids (mg)	Carotenoids (mcg or mg)	PE (mcg or mg)	Folate (mcg)	Selenium (mcg)	Vit. C (mg)	Vit. E (IUs)
Peas and onions	½ cup	41	0.2/0	2	na	189 mcg (BC)	na	18	0.4	6	0.15
Peas and potatoes	½ cup	67	0.1/0	3	na	144 mcg (BC)	na	29	0.9	9	0.3
Ratatouille	½ cup	76	6/0.8	2	na	179 mcg (BC)	na	14	0.5	10	1.4
Succotash	½ cup	89	0.9/0.2	4	na	132 mcg (BC)	na	32	0.6	6	0.45
Summer squash and onions	½ cup	27	0.2/0	1	na	102 mcg (BC)	na	17	0.3	5	0.15
Vegetable and pasta combination	½ cup	90	4/1	0.6	na	1.5 mg (BC)	na	18	3	9	0.3
Vegetables, stew type	½ cup	39	0.1/0	2	na	3 mg (BC)	na	10	0.4	5	0.3
Vegetable stir fry	½ cup	34	0.05/0	1	na	na	na	na	na	23	na
Zucchini w/ tomato sauce	½ cup	20	0.1/0	2	na	269 mcg (BC)	na	15	0.5	10	0.3

YOGURT

Food	Serving Size	Calories	Fat/Sat. Fat (gm)	Fiber (gm)	Flavonoids (mg)	Carotenoids (mcg or mg)	PE (mcg or mg)	Folate (mcg)	Selenium (mcg)	Vit. C (mg)	Vit. E (IUs)
Yogurt, lowfat:											
Fruit flavored	1 cup	250	2.6/1.7	0	0	15 mcg (BC)	0	23	7.6	1.6	0.15
Plain	1 cup	155	3.8/2.5	0	0	29 mcg (BC)	0	27	8	2	0.15
Vanilla, lemon, or coffee	1 cup	209	3/2	0	0	15 mcg (BC)	0	26	12	1.8	0.15
Yogurt, nonfat:											
Fruit flavored	1 cup	230	0.5/0.3	0	0	0	0	22	15	1.7	0
Fruit flavored (sugar free)	1 cup	122	0.4/0.2	0	0	15 mcg (BC)	0	32	7	26	0.3
Plain	1 cup	137	0.4/0.3	0	0	0	0	30	9	2	0
Vanilla, lemon, or coffee	1 cup	223	0.4/0.3	0	0	0	0	27	8	2	0
Vanilla, lemon, or coffee (sugar free)	1 cup	105	0.4/0.3	0	0	0	0	20	7.6	2.7	0.15

Food	Serving Size	Calories	Fat/Sat. Fat (gm)	Fiber (gm)	Flavonoids (mg)	Carotenoids (mcg or mg)	PE (mcg or mg)	Folate (mcg)	Selenium (mcg)	Vit. C (mg)	Vit. E (IUs)
Yogurt, whole milk:											
Fruit flavored	1 cup	291	8/5	0	0	47 mcg (BC)	0	22	7.4	1.6	0.3
Plain	1 cup	150.5	8/5	0	0	44 mcg (BC)	0	18	5.4	1.3	0.3
Vanilla, lemon, or coffee	1 cup	247	8/5	0	0	44 mcg (BC)	0	25	12	1.8	0.3

REFERENCES

Chapter 1: Resist Cancer Now

American Cancer Society. 2002. The complete guide—nutrition and physical activity. Online: www.cancer.org

American Institute for Cancer Research. 2002. Food, nutrition and the prevention of cancer: a global perspective. Online: www.aicr.org

American Institute for Cancer Research. 2002. Simple steps to prevent cancer. Online: www.aicr.org

Cancer Research Foundation of America. 2002. Women's health—diet. Online: www.preventcancer.org

Editor. 1999. Vitamins, carotenoids, and phytochemicals. Online: www.webmd.com

Lewis, C. J., et al. 1999. Health claims and observational data: relation between dietary fat and cancer. *American Journal of Clinical Nutrition* 69:1357S–1364S.

McCord, H. 1996. Savor the new white-hot superfood. *Prevention.* January, 79–83.

Messina, M., et al. 2002. Gaining insight into the health effects of soy but a long way still to go: commentary on the

Fourth International Symposium on the role of soy in preventing and treating chronic disease. *Journal of Nutrition* 132:547S–551S.

Nijveldt, R. J. 2001. Flavonoids: a review of probable mechanisms of action and potential applications. *American Journal of Clinical Nutrition* 74:418–425.

Steinmetz, K. A., et al. 1996. Vegetables, fruit, and cancer prevention: a review. *Journal of the American Dietetic Association* 96:1027–1039.

Webb, D. 1997. The real cancer miracle. *Prevention.* March, pp. 92–96.

Willett, W. C. 2000. Diet and cancer. *The Oncologist* 5:393–404.

Yang, C. S., et al. 2001. Inhibition of carcinogenesis by dietary polyphenolic compounds. *Annual Review of Nutrition* 21:381–406.

Chapter 2: From Market to Meals: Maximize the Anti-Cancer Power of Your Food

Applegate, L. 1996. Going organic. *Runner's World.* August, pp. 30–31.

Clark, N. 1996. Healthy cooking: There's no place like home. *The Physician and Sportsmedicine.* February. Online: www.physsportsmed.com

Editor. 2001. Canned vegetables aren't all bad. *Countryside & Small Stock Journal.* November, p. 50.

Editor. 1997. Fill your plate and lose weight. *Prevention.* February, pp. 104–105.

Editor. 1995. Keep summer alive in your freezer. *Consumers' Research Magazine.* August, pp. 28–32.

Editor. 1998. Organic foods: sure root to health? *Health Quest.* October 31, p. 25.

Gutfeld, G. 1998. This little pig goes to market. *Men's Health.* June, pp. 150–157.

Kleiner, S. M. 2001. *Power eating.* Champaign, Illinois: Human Kinetics Publishers.

Marion, M. 1998. The vegetable hater's guide to nutrition. *Men's Health.* March, pp. 72–74.

Mather, M. 1996. Eating fresh all year round. *Mother Earth News.* August 18, pp. 42–50.

McCord, H. et al. 1999. 5 great cooking tips for the healthiest meat. *Prevention.* April, p. 60.

Nagle, M., et al. 1995. Superfood: oatmeal. *Prevention.* October 10, pp. 140–141.

Olney, J., et al. 1994. Summer fresh-fruit finales. *Prevention.* July, pp. 98–111.

Organic Trade Association. 2002. Ten good reasons to buy organic. Online: www.ota.com

Segal, M. 1988. Fruit: something food that's not illegal, immortal, or fattening. *FDA Consumer.* May, pp. 10–13.

Webb, D. 1997. The real cancer miracle. *Prevention.* March, pp. 92–96.

Chapter 3: The 10-Step Anti-Cancer Diet

American Cancer Society. 2002. The complete guide—nutrition and physical activity. Online: www.cancer.org

American Institute for Cancer Research. 2002. Simple steps to prevent cancer. Online: www.aicr.org

Barr, S. I. 1999. Cancer-fighting foods. *Bicycling.* May, pp. 48–49.

Carper, J. 1995. *Stop aging now!* New York: HarperCollins Publishers.

Editor. 1998. Dairy foods may reduce colon cancer risk. *Business Wire,* September 21.

McCord, H. 2001. Polish up some cancer protection. *Prevention.* October, p. 67.

Murray, M. T. 1996. *Encyclopedia of nutritional substances.* Rocklin, California.

Ochs, R. 1997. Vitamin role in cancer? Daily intake, sun may lower risk. *Newsday.* November 2, p. A31.

Recer, T. 2002. Study: Calcium may lower cancer risk. Associated Press, March 19.

Thomas, H. 2001. Foods can reduce the risk of breast cancer. *The London Free Press.* August 8, p. C3.

Webb, D. 1999. Do you need a dose of "good" bacteria? *Prevention.* May, pp. 65–66.

Yang, C. S., et al. 2001. Inhibition of carcinogenesis by dietary polyphenolic compounds. *Annual Review of Nutrition* 21:381–406.

Chapter 5: The Anti-Cancer Nutrition Counter

Beecher, G. R. 1998. Nutrient content of tomatoes and tomato products. *Proceedings of the Society for Experimental Biology and Medicine* 218:98–100.

Dwyer, J. T., et al. 1994. Tofu and soy drinks contain phytoestrogens. *Journal of the American Dietetic Association* 94:739–743.

Franke, A., et al. 1999. Isoflavone levels in soy foods consumed by multiethnic populations in Singapore and Hawaii. *Journal of Agriculture and Food Chemistry* 47:977–986.

Lapcik, O., et al. 1998. Identification of isoflavones in beer. *Steroids* 63:14–20.

Liggins, J., et al. 2000a. Daidzen and genistein content of fruits and nuts. *The Journal of Nutritional Biochemistry* 11:326–331.

———2000b. Daidzen and genistein content of vegetables. *The British Journal of Nutrition* 84:717–725.

Mazur, W. M. 1998. Phytoestrogen content in foods. *Balliere's Clinical Endocrinology and Metabolism* 12: 729–742.

Mazur, W. M., et al. 2000. Phytoestrogen content of berries, and plasma concentrations and urinary excretion of enterolactone after a single strawberry-meal in human subjects. *The British Journal of Nutrition* 83:381–387.

Nair, S., et al. 1998. Antioxidant phenolics and flavonoids in common Indian foods. *The Journal of the Association of Physicians of India* 46:708–710.

Nutrient Data Laboratory. USDA Nutrient Database for Standard Reference, Release 13; USDA Nutrient Database for Standard Reference, Release 14. Beltsville, Maryland: U.S. Department of Agriculture.

Reinli, K., et al. 1996. Phytoestrogen content of foods—a compendium of literature values. *Nutrition and Cancer* 26:123–148.

Ross, S. A., et al. 2000. Variance of common flavonoids by brand of grapefruit juice. *Fitoterapia* 71:154–161.

Scalbert, A., et al. 2000. Dietary intake and bioavailability of polyphenols. *The Journal of Nutrition.* 130:2073S–2085S.

Setchell, K. D., et al. Bioavailability of pure isoflavones in healthy humans and analysis of commercial soy isoflavone supplements. *Journal of Nutrition* 131:1362S–1375S.

U.S. Department of Agriculture. 1998. Carotenoid database for U.S. foods.

U.S. Department of Agriculture-Iowa State University. 1999. Database for the isoflavone content of foods.

Vinson, J., et al. 2001. Phenol antioxidant quantity and quality in foods: fruits. *Journal of Agriculture and Food Chemistry* 49:5315–5321.